Aromatherapy

ESSENTIAL OILS IN COLOUR

Caddy Classic Profiles

by Rosemary Caddy
BSc ARCS MISPA

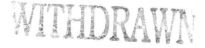
Published by
Amberwood Publishing Ltd
Rochester, Kent ME2 4HU
books@amberwoodpublishing.com

© Amberwood Publishing Ltd 1997

First Edition June 1997
Second Edition April 2000
Reprinted December 2001
Reprinted February 2005

© Authors Copyright Rosemary Caddy 1997

ISBN 1 899308 14 8

Cover design by Howland Northover & Rosemary Caddy

Printed in China

CONTENTS

Oil List

1	AMYRIS	Amyris balsamifera	Rutaceae
2	BASIL EUGENOL	Ocimum gratissimum eug.	Lamiaceae
3	BASIL EXOTIC REUNION	Ocimum basilicum	Lamiaceae
4	BASIL SWEET EUROPEAN	Ocimum basilicum	Lamiaceae
5	BASIL THYMOL	Ocimum gratissimum thym.	Lamiaceae
6	BENZOIN	Styrax benzoin	Styracaceae
7	BERGAMOT	Citrus bergamia	Rutaceae
8	BLACK PEPPER	Piper nigrum	Piperaceae
9	CADE	Juniperus oxycedrus	Cupressaceae
10	CARAWAY SEED	Carum carvi	Umbelliferae
11	CARROT SEED	Daucus carota	Umbelliferae
12	CATNIP	Nepata cataria	Lamiaceae
13	CEDAR TEXAS	Juniperus ashei	Cupressaceae
14	CEDAR VIRGINIAN RED	Juniperus virginiana	Cupressaceae
15	CEDARWOOD ATLAS	Cedrus atlantica	Pinaceae
16	CHAMOMILE GERMAN	Matricaria recutica	Compositae
17	CHAMOMILE MAROC	Ormenis multicaulis	Compositae
18	CHAMOMILE ROMAN	Chamaemelum nobile	Compositae
19	CINNAMON LEAF	Cinnamomum zeylanicum	Lauraceae
20	CLARY SAGE	Salvia sclarea	Lamiaceae
21	CLOVE BUD	Syzygium aromaticum	Myrtaceae
22	CORIANDER	Coriandrum sativum	Umbelliferae
23	CYPRESS	Cupressus sempervirens	Cupressaceae
24	DILL	Anethum graveolens	Umbelliferae
25	EUCALYPTUS BLUE GUM	Eucalyptus globulus	Myrtaceae
26	EUCALYPTUS DIVES	Eucalyptus dives	Myrtaceae
27	EUCALYPTUS LEMON SC.	Eucalyptus citriodora	Myrtaceae
28	EUCALYPTUS SMITHII	Eucalyptus smithii	Myrtaceae
29	EUCALYPTUS STAIGERIANA	Eucalyptus staigeriana	Myrtaceae
30	FENNEL SWEET	Foeniculum vulgare	Umbelliferae
31	FIR NEEDLE SILVER	Abies alba	Pinaceae
32	FRANKINCENSE	Boswellia carteri	Buseraceae
33	GERANIUM	Pelargonium graveolens	Geraniaceae
34	GINGER	Zingiber officinale	Zingiberaceae
35	GRAPEFRUIT	Citrus paradisi	Rutaceae
36	HYSSOP	Hyssopus officinalis	Lamiaceae
37	JASMIN	Jasminum officinale	Oleaceae
38	JUNIPER BERRY	Juniperus communis	Cupressaceae
39	JUNIPER TWIGS	Juniperus communis	Cupressaceae
40	LAVANDIN	Lavandula hybrida	Lamiaceae
41	LAVENDER SPIKE	Lavandula lactifolia	Lamiaceae
42	LAVENDER TRUE	Lavandula angustifolia	Lamiaceae
43	LEMON	Citrus limon	Rutaceae
44	LEMONGRASS EAST INDIAN	Cymbopogon flexuosus	Gramineae
45	LEMONGRASS WEST INDIAN	Cymbopogon citratus	Gramineae

Oil List

46	LIME	Citrus aurantifolia	Rutaceae
47	MANDARIN	Citrus reticulata	Rutaceae
48	MARJORAM SPANISH	Thymus mastichina	Lamiaceae
49	MARJORAM SWEET	Origanum majorana	Lamiaceae
50	MELISSA LEMON BALM	Melissa officinalis	Lamiaceae
51	MINT BERGAMOT	Mentha citrata	Lamiaceae
52	MINT CORNMINT	Mentha arvensis	Lamiaceae
53	MINT PEPPERMINT	Mentha piperita	Lamiaceae
54	MINT SPEARMINT	Mentha spicata	Lamiaceae
55	MYRRH	Commiphora molmol	Buseraceae
56	NIAOULI	Melaleuca viridiflora	Myrtaceae
57	NUTMEG	Myristica fragrans	Myristicaceae
58	ORANGE BITTER	Citrus aurantium amara	Rutaceae
59	ORANGE BLOSSOM NEROLI	Citrus aurantium amara	Rutaceae
60	ORANGE PETITGRAIN	Citrus aurantium amara	Rutaceae
61	ORANGE SWEET	Citrus sinensis	Rutaceae
62	OREGANUM	Origanum hera. carvacroliferum	Lamiaceae
63	PALMAROSA	Cymbopogon martinii	Gramineae
64	PATCHOULI	Pogostemon cablin	Lamiaceae
65	PENNYROYAL	Mentha pulegium	Lamiaceae
66	PINE DWARF	Pinus mugo turra	Pinaceae
67	PINE LONGLEAF TURP.	Pinus palustris	Pinaceae
68	PINE LONGLEAF WOOD	Pinus palustris	Pinaceae
69	PINE SCOTCH	Pinus sylvestris	Pinaceae
70	RAVENSARA AROMATIC	Ravensara aromatica	Lauraceae
71	ROSE OTTO	Rosa damascena	Rosaceae
72	ROSEMARY	Rosmarinus officinalis	Lamiaceae
73	ROSEWOOD	Aniba rosaeodora	Lauraceae
74	SAGE COMMON	Salvia officinalis	Lamiaceae
75	SAGE SPANISH	Salvia lavendulaefolia	Lamiaceae
76	SANDALWOOD	Santalum album	Santalaceae
77	SAVORY SUMMER	Satureja hortensis	Lamiaceae
78	SAVORY WINTER	Satureja montana	Lamiaceae
79	SPRUCE CANADIAN BLACK	Picea mariana nigra	Pinaceae
80	SPRUCE HEMLOCK	Tsuga canadensis	Pinaceae
81	TAGETES	Tagetes glandulifera	Compositae
82	TARRAGON	Artemisia dracunculus	Compositae
83	TEATREE	Melaleuca alternifolia	Myrtaceae
84	THUJA WHITE CEDAR	Thuja occidentalis	Cupressaceae
85	THYME COMMON RED/WH.	Thymus vulgaris thymoliferum	Lamiaceae
86	THYME COMMON SWEET	Thymus vulgaris linalol/geraniol	Lamiaceae
87	THYME MOROCCAN	Thymus satureioides	Lamiaceae
88	VETIVER	Vetiveria zizanoides	Gramineae
89	YARROW	Achillea millefolium	Compositae
90	YLANG YLANG	Cananga odorata	Annonaceae

About the Author

Rosemary Caddy, BSc Hons, ARCS, MISPA

Rosemary Caddy graduated from London University with a BSc Honours Degree in Science. As a Reader and Principal Lecturer in Educational Research at Nottingham University she is the author of a range of educational materials for students of many disciplines. All the materials emphasise visual presentation to enable students to see, analyse and understand the world around them. The format of this work ranges from books to interactive video tapes and compact discs.

Rosemary is now a qualified clinical aromatherapist running her own clinic and carrying out a programme of research on the chemistry of essential oils. She runs lecture courses for aromatherapy students to help them understand and visualise their essential oils. The Caddy Classic Profiles, developed as a result of her research enable students to enjoy the chemistry of their oils.

Currently Rosemary is researching the chemistry of synergistic mixes of essential oils.

Acknowledgements

My interest in essential oils derives from personal experience of their powerful therapeutic properties, both in treating physical ailments and also in calming emotional problems.

Exploring the chemistry of essential oils gives some insights as to why the oils are so powerful.

My background in lecturing and research has been focused on using strong visual stumuli to communicate complex structures. Colour and pictures are excellent learning aids. Caddy Classic Profiles have been created to help communicate the nature of essential oils.

I would like to sincerely thank the following people who have contributed to this book in a variety of ways: John Ensall for his support since the early days to develop my ideas and for generous sharing of chemical data; Elaine Price of the Montrose School of Massage and Aromatherapy who recognised the work in its first stages and encouraged me to write the book offering many valuable suggestions; Katja Svoboda and her team at The Scottish Agricultural College for assistance in research into essential oils and their synergistic mixes; and Henry Crisp together with the Amberwood production team for the publication of the book.

I would also like to thank all my friends, family, colleagues and students who listened to all my enthusiasms so patiently. In particular special thanks to Peter, my husband, for his unflagging support and for his painstaking editing of manuscript and indices.

My appreciation also goes to the services of Nottingham and Exeter University Libraries, The British Library, The Royal Horticultural Society, Oxford Botanical Gardens and to my own local Dartmouth Library.

It is my hope that this book will offer the opportunity to the reader to build an understanding of each essential oil in a pleasurable but powerful way.

Note to the Reader

Whilst the author has made every effort to ensure that the contents of this book are accurate in every particular, it is not intended to be regarded as a substitute for professional medical advice under treatment. The reader is urged to give careful consideration to any difficulties which he or she is experiencing with their own health and to consult their General Practitioner if uncertain as to its cause or nature. Neither the author nor the publisher can accept any legal responsibility for any health problem which results from use of the self-help methods described.

1 | An Introduction to Caddy Profiles and Caddy Classic Profiles

1 | Essential Oils

Essential oils are products of a plant's metabolic processes. Each plant stores this oil in different parts of its structure. The oil may be found in the petals, leaves, twigs, fruit, wood, bark, roots and other areas. Methods by which the oil is extracted from the plant vary according to its distribution in the plant. Steam distillation is the commonest extraction technique for essential oils. Extraction by expression is used for many of the citrus oils. Other methods include enfleurage, solvent extraction and carbon dioxide extraction. Strangely enough an essential oil is not used by its plant in fact it appears to be 'non essential' to the plant - the name essential oil means that it is an oil that is volatile at room temperature. Thus in use it evaporates leaving no trace. The oils that evaporate most quickly are referred to as 'top note' oils, those with very slow evaporation rates are referred to as 'base note' oils and those with evaporation rates in between are referred to as 'middle note' oils. The 'note' of the oil is very important when blending oils in particular for the perfumer. Essential oils have aromas ranging from earthy herbal tones to light floral tones and have been used to heal the body and spirit since ancient times.

This book reports the widely accepted therapeutic properties and uses of ninety essential oils. The properties and uses are related to the major body systems - nervous system, endocrine system, circulation and immune system, skin, muscles and body tissues, respiratory system, digestive system, urinary system and reproductive system.

The chemical make up of an essential oil is important. Due to the fact that an oil may well have hundreds of chemical constituents it is a challenge to communicate its chemical nature. Caddy Profiles have been created to meet this challenge. A Caddy Profile gives a simple and immediate colour picture of an oil. The following section gives you a full description of a Caddy Profile followed with notes on how it was developed.

A Caddy Profile will help you to see the chemical nature of an oil at a glance. It also communicates the expected therapeutic nature of the oil. It allows you to compare it with other oils and can also alert you to possible adulteration of an oil.

A Caddy Profile gives a 'finger print' of the oil - a visual memory of the oil that has not been available before.

Introduction to Caddy Profiles

LAVENDER TRUE OIL

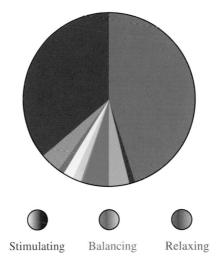

Stimulating   Balancing   Relaxing

Caddy Profiles will help to enhance your understanding of the nature of the oils and also give a simple means of comparing their properties. To introduce the concept of such a profile we work carefully through two examples building up the information contained in a profile step by step. The first example to be considered is Lavender True.

Lavender True *(lavandula angustifolia)*
Lavender oil is known to be helpful in treating a wide range of problems. It is the number one choice for the first aid kit at home. It relaxes you if you are tense and stimulates you when you are low. It can heal burns and deal with headaches. It soothes inflamed joints and helps you to sleep and so on and so on. Why is it such a powerful yet gentle healing agent?

Look at the Caddy Profile for lavender.
The yellow through to red colours indicate the presence of stimulating properties in an oil whereas the blue colours indicate the presence of relaxing properties. The green colours indicate neither relaxing nor stimulating properties and are thus referred to as balancing colours.

The words 'stimulating', 'balancing' and 'relaxing' are used here in a general sense. 'Stimulating' suggests enlivening or triggering. 'Balancing' suggests regulating. 'Relaxing' suggests calming, release of tension and stress.

In lavender the Caddy Profile shows:

- large areas of both blue and red.

This indicates that lavender oil can be both relaxing and stimulating. It is well known that lavender oil does indeed reflect this indication in that it relaxes you when you are tense and stimulates you when you are low.

- ten different colours.

This indicates that lavender oil will have a wide set of properties relating to these colours that will make it effective for many different conditions.

TEA TREE OIL

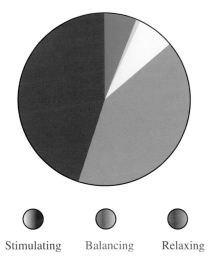

Stimulating   Balancing   Relaxing

Tea Tree *(melaleuca alternifolia)*

For a second example consider tea tree oil. This again is a well known oil. It has strong antiseptic and antifungal properties. It is excellent for clearing congestion and is a strong stimulant to the system.

The Caddy Profile above shows:

- over 90% of the area is coloured by yellow to red. This indicates that tea tree oil is highly stimulating.

- five different colours. This indicates that tea tree oil may not have as wide a range of applications as lavender.

The Colours and the Chemical Families

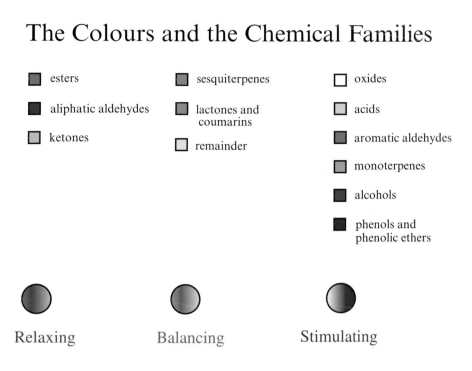

- esters
- aliphatic aldehydes
- ketones

- sesquiterpenes
- lactones and coumarins
- remainder

- oxides
- acids
- aromatic aldehydes
- monoterpenes
- alcohols
- phenols and phenolic ethers

Relaxing   Balancing   Stimulating

EACH COLOUR USED IN A CADDY PROFILE REPRESENTS A CHEMICAL FAMILY

By just the two examples given it is clear that Caddy Profiles communicate the nature of oils and give the opportunity to compare oils visually. However once we explore the meaning of the individual colours the profiles become even more useful. Essential oils are made up of hundreds of chemical constituents. The majority of these constituents can be grouped into the eleven chemical families listed above.

Research by Pierre Franchomme (see later) suggests that the chemical families can be clustered into these groups according to their electrochemical behaviour. Caddy profiles always place the chemical families in the same order with 'blues' suggesting first type of behaviour, 'greens' suggesting the second type of behaviour, and 'yellow through to red' suggesting the third type of behaviour.

LAVENDER TRUE
Lavandula angustifolia

■	esters	45.0%
■	aliphatic aldehydes	1.0%
☐	ketones	4.0%
■	sesquiterpenes	5.0%
■	lactones and coumarins	0.3%
☐	remainder	1.7%
☐	oxides	2.0%
■	aromatic aldehydes	1.0%
■	monoterpenes	4.0%
■	alcohols	36.0%
■	phenols,phe. ethers	yes

Stimulating   Balancing   Relaxing

If you always read the list of chemical families from top to bottom and read the Profile from '12 o'clock' in a clockwise direction you will start with the most relaxing family and end up with the most stimulating family in the oil. Now that we have the list of chemical families in lavender we can expand on the information that its Caddy Profile gives us:

■ - containing a large proportion of esters, lavender will exhibit the properties of esters i.e. effective healing of wounds and scars, cooling and anti-inflammatory help for skin disorders...

■ ■ - both types of aldehydes are present in small amounts - likely to be only beneficial with no sensitisation problems...

☐ - ketones to help congestion...

☐ - oxides provide help for respiratory problems...

■ - monoterpenes offer antiviral properties amongst others...

■ - the large proportion of alcohols indicates that lavender will have good stimulating properties that act in a powerful but gentle manner...

TEA TREE
Melaleuca alternifolia

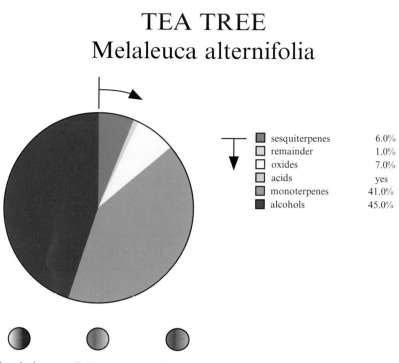

■	sesquiterpenes	6.0%
□	remainder	1.0%
□	oxides	7.0%
□	acids	yes
■	monoterpenes	41.0%
■	alcohols	45.0%

Stimulating   Balancing   Relaxing

For a final illustration consider the properties of tea tree as indicated by its chemical make up shown above:

■ - containing sesquiterpenes indicates amongst others antiseptic and antispasmodic actions...

□ - the oxides indicate a good agent for the respiratory system...

■ - containing a large proportion of monoterpenes tea tree will exhibit bactericidal and antiviral properties, be a good expectorant and stimulating to the nervous system...

■ - containing a large proportion of alcohols indicates again powerful stimulation, also antifungal and bactericidal properties...

The chapter 'Body Systems and Therapeutic Properties of the Chemical Families' gives you full information on possible therapeutic properties of each chemical family related to the major systems of the body. This allows you to compare known properties of each oil with its chemical make up and its possible therapeutic uses in a way not easily accessible before.

This book presents the Caddy Classic Profiles (see later) for ninety oils together with guiding notes on their nature, their botanical heritage and their therapeutic properties.

Note from the author - How I Developed the Idea of Caddy Profiles.

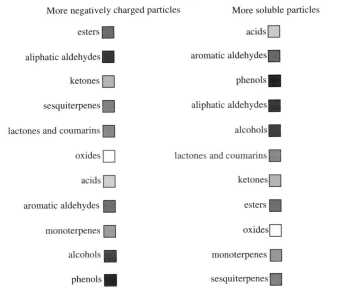

More negatively charged particles

esters	■
aliphatic aldehydes	■
ketones	□
sesquiterpenes	■
lactones and coumarins	■
oxides	□
acids	□
aromatic aldehydes	■
monoterpenes	■
alcohols	■
phenols	■

More positively charged particles

More soluble particles

acids	□
aromatic aldehydes	■
phenols	■
aliphatic aldehydes	■
alcohols	■
lactones and coumarins	■
ketones	■
esters	■
oxides	□
monoterpenes	■
sesquiterpenes	■

Less soluble particles

Pierre Franchomme's research reports an experiment where molecules of chemical constituents are sprayed between two electromagnetic plates. Negatively charged particles are attracted to the positive plate and positively charged particles are attracted to the negative plate. Interestingly the particles cluster into the chemical families.

The experiment reports both the solubility and magnetic attraction of the particles. Both of these characteristics are important when considering the nature of each chemical constituent. The two columns above suggest an ordering of the families against the two characteristics as shown by the experiment.

Franchomme and colleagues have carried out many clinical experiments in French hospitals exploring the importance of the electrochemical nature of molecules.

Franchomme's clinical work suggests that negatively charged particles appear in general to have more relaxing effects compared to more stimulating effects of the positively charged particles. This might be due to the negatively charged particles tending to donate electrons and the positively charged particles tending to accept electrons. Uncharged particles are likely to be more stable.

I decided to explore this idea over ninety oils with this book being the result.

First of all I allocated colours in the following way. In the experiment esters, aliphatic aldehydes and ketones appear to generate more negative particles - these families are coloured in shades of blue. Sesquiterpenes, lactones and coumarins appear to generate more neutral particles - these families are coloured in shades of green. Oxides, acids, aromatic aldehydes, monoterpenes, alcohols and phenols appear to generate more positive particles these families are coloured yellow through to red. Given the chemical constituents in an oil I could now draw a Caddy Profile.

As suggested by the examples of tea tree and lavender the colour coding proves to be a useful general guide to the nature of all the oils. As well as Franchomme's ideas on the stimulating and relaxing properties being linked to the electrochemical nature of a chemical constituent other observations emerge from examining the ninety oils. Certain sesquiterpenols and aromatic alcohols, due to their molecular size and structure, may exhibit calming properties. This is apparent in amyris, sandalwood and rose oils. Oils such as the cold pressed citrus oils, that are mainly monoterpenes, exhibit a calming and cheering nature. Another useful aspect of the colour coding is that it alerts you immediately to the presence of ketones and phenols. Any oil with a large percentage of either of these families needs to be used with care. Ketones can be powerful and they may also accumulate in the body. Phenols can be highly aggressive.

This book provides you with:

1   The properties and uses, as reported by practitioners, of each oil.

2   The chemical make-up of each oil colour coded as a Caddy Profile which shows at a glance its chemical nature. Also all the major individual chemical constituents are listed.

3   A list of the chemical families with suggestions of possible properties that may occur if they are present in an oil.

Using this book you can explore how the known properties of your oils relate to their chemical makeup. Chemical constituents are likely to exhibit some but not all their possible family properties. It is rare for them not to exhibit any family properties. Also remember that each oil is unique and must be considered as a whole. The chemical constituents in an oil often enhance each other (synergy) and can occasionally oppose each other (antagonism).

Each of your clients brings a new set of variables and you need to be aware of the personal relationship between your client and the oils. The structured layout of all the information in this book will help you make informed choices of oils.

Body Systems and Therapeutic Properties of the Chemical Families

This chapter gives therapeutic notes on each of the eleven major chemical families that are shown in Caddy Profiles. This enables you to build up a picture of the therapeutic properties of any of the oils in the book. This is made easier by classifying the properties against major systems of the body. The body systems are always listed in the order below.

NERVOUS SYSTEM

This is the major control system of the body. It includes the brain, spinal column and all the network of nerves that carry both the conscious and subconscious signals to all parts of the body. It controls all life support functions and conveys all information received from external and internal stimuli around the body .

ENDOCRINE SYSTEM

This is the glandular system of the body. It feeds back information as to the current state of the body and triggers the release of hormones to instruct the body to change state. For example the pituitary gland monitors the menstrual cycle and releases hormones appropriately. There are many feedback mechanisms of this nature. The endocrine system is also very much a control system hence it has been placed next in order to the nervous system.

CIRCULATION AND IMMUNE SYSTEM

These consist of the blood network and the lympth network. These networks deliver raw materials to all parts of the body and also collect all the waste products. The immune system is made up of cells that are carried in these networks. The cells have the capacity to defend the body against malfunction due to intruders such as bacteria and viruses.

SKIN, MUSCLE AND BODY TISSUES

This system includes the skin (which is the single largest organ of the body with many protective and controlling functions) , the soft connective tissues, the muscles and the skeleton of the body. All the members of this system physically support the body as well as performing other wide ranging processes. Muscles obviously control physical movements in response to signals from the nervous system. Bones support the body and bone marrow manufactures new blood cells and so on. Indeed all the systems of the body are interacting continuously. This classification is just to structure our thoughts to help in building up profiles of the effects of the oils.

RESPIRATORY SYSTEM

This system consists of the air passages and lungs. It is responsible for providing the blood system with oxygen to deliver to all parts of the body and for extracting the carbon dioxide from the blood when it returns to the lungs.

DIGESTIVE SYSTEM

This system is responsible for processing food so that the blood system can deliver it to all parts of the body in an appropriate form. The alimentary canal links to many organs of the body each of which is programmed to process the food in certain ways. In the mouth the enzymes start breaking the food down. In the stomach hydrochloric acid takes action. The liver is responsible for complex food processing and so on and so on right through the alimentary canal until the waste products are excreted through the rectum.

URINARY SYSTEM

This system consists of the kidneys and the urethrae. The kidneys are responsible for filtering the waste products out of the blood which is excreted as urine. The kidneys carry a major responsibility for the health of the blood.

REPRODUCTIVE SYSTEM

This system consists of all the male and female reproductive organs. The functioning of these is closely linked to the hormones released through the endocrine system.

The Chemical Families

Individual chemical constituents may exhibit some of the characteristics of the chemical family they belong to.

 Esters

NERVOUS SYSTEM
- antispasmodic, calming, cheering, healing, uplifting

ENDOCRINE SYSTEM
- balancing

CIRCULATION AND IMMUNE SYSTEM
- calming

SKIN, MUSCLE AND BODY TISSUES
- antifungal, antiinflammatory, cell regenerator, soothing for rashes, good for scar tissue, vulnerary

RESPIRATORY SYSTEM
- antiinflammatory, antispasmodic

DIGESTIVE SYSTEM
- antiinflammatory, calming

URINARY SYSTEM
- antiinflammatory, calming

REPRODUCTIVE SYSTEM
- calming

Esters are generally gentle and safe in nature. They are a good choice for treating the young, old or frail.

Aliphatic Aldehydes

NERVOUS SYSTEM
- calming

ENDOCRINE SYSTEM
- temperature reducing

CIRCULATION AND IMMUNE SYSTEM
- antiviral, lowers blood pressure

SKIN, MUSCLE AND BODY TISSUES
- antifungal, antiinflammatory, antiseptic, irritant

RESPIRATORY SYSTEM
- antiseptic, antiviral

DIGESTIVE SYSTEM
- antiseptic, antiviral

URINARY SYSTEM
- antiseptic, antiviral

REPRODUCTIVE SYSTEM
- antiseptic, antiviral

Ketones

NERVOUS SYSTEM
- analgesic, calming, sedative, uplifting

ENDOCRINE SYSTEM
- stimulates secretions, cooling

CIRCULATION AND IMMUNE SYSTEM
- anticoagulant, decongestant

SKIN, MUSCLE AND BODY TISSUES
- antifungal, antiinflammatory, parasiticide, good for scar tissue

☐ Ketones (continued)

RESPIRATORY SYSTEM
- mucolytic, expectorant

DIGESTIVE SYSTEM
- aids liver function, breaks down fats

URINARY SYSTEM
- antifungal, antiinflammatory

REPRODUCTIVE SYSTEM
- decongestant, emmenagogue

Ketones should be used with care as they can build up in the body.

■ Sesquiterpenes

NERVOUS SYSTEM
- slightly analgesic, antispasmodic, calming, relaxes cramps

ENDOCRINE SYSTEM
- balancing

CIRCULATION AND IMMUNE SYSTEM
- astringent, bactericidal, slightly reduces blood pressure

SKIN, MUSCLE AND BODY TISSUES
- antifungal, antiinflammatory, antiseptic

RESPIRATORY SYSTEM
- antiseptic, bactericidal, balancing

DIGESTIVE SYSTEM
- antiseptic, bactericidal, balancing

URINARY SYSTEM
- antiseptic, bactericidal, balancing

REPRODUCTIVE SYSTEM
- antiseptic, bactericidal, balancing

■ Lactones and Coumarins

NERVOUS SYSTEM
- calming, sedative, uplifting

ENDOCRINE SYSTEM
- increases sweating, reduces temperature

CIRCULATION AND IMMUNE SYSTEM
- anticoagulant, lowers blood pressure, decongestant

SKIN, MUSCLE AND BODY TISSUES
- can be phototoxic

RESPIRATORY SYSTEM
- mucolytic, decongestant, relieves catarrh

DIGESTIVE SYSTEM
- balancing

URINARY SYSTEM
- balancing

REPRODUCTIVE SYSTEM
- balancing

☐ Oxides

NERVOUS SYSTEM
- stimulant

ENDOCRINE SYSTEM
- stimulates secretions particularly from the pancreas

CIRCULATION AND IMMUNE SYSTEM
- anticoagulant, decongestant

SKIN, MUSCLE AND BODY TISSUES
- can be irritant

☐ Oxides (continued)

RESPIRATORY SYSTEM
- expectorant, decongestant, mucolytic

DIGESTIVE SYSTEM
- stimulant

URINARY SYSTEM
- diuretic

REPRODUCTIVE SYSTEM
- stimulant

☐ Acids

SKIN, MUSCLE AND BODY TISSUES
- antiinflammatory, deodorant

Generally organic acids occur only in small quantities. They react chemically with alcohols to form esters and water.

■ Aromatic Aldehydes

NERVOUS SYSTEM
- calming

ENDOCRINE SYSTEM
- reduces temperature

CIRCULATION AND IMMUNE SYSTEM
- antiviral, lowers blood pressure

SKIN, MUSCLE AND BODY TISSUES
- antifungal, antiinflammatory, antiseptic, irritant

RESPIRATORY SYSTEM
- antiseptic, antiviral

DIGESTIVE SYSTEM
- antiseptic, antiviral

URINARY SYSTEM
- antiseptic, antiviral

REPRODUCTIVE SYSTEM
- antiseptic, antiviral

These are the same properties as the aliphatic aldehydes but the aromatic aldehydes are generally more stimulating and warming.

■ Monoterpenes

NERVOUS SYSTEM
- slightly analgesic, stimulant

ENDOCRINE SYSTEM
- stimulates secretions particularly bile, liver and gall bladder

CIRCULATION AND IMMUNE SYSTEM
- antiviral, bactericidal, decongestant

SKIN, MUSCLE AND BODY TISSUES
- air antiseptic

RESPIRATORY SYSTEM
- antiviral, bactericidal, expectorant

DIGESTIVE SYSTEM
- decongestant, breaks down gall stones

URINARY SYSTEM
- antiviral, bactericidal, decongestant

REPRODUCTIVE SYSTEM
- antiviral, bactericidal, decongestant

■ Alcohols

NERVOUS SYSTEM
- stimulant, good tonic, uplifting, warming

ENDOCRINE SYSTEM
- balancing, hormone like, stimulates secretions

CIRCULATION AND IMMUNE SYSTEM
- antiviral, strongly bactericidal, decongestant, may lower blood pressure particularly sesquiterpenols

SKIN, MUSCLE AND BODY TISSUES
- antifungal, antiseptic, free from irritation

RESPIRATORY SYSTEM
- antiviral, bactericidal

DIGESTIVE SYSTEM
- stimulant, warming

URINARY SYSTEM
- diuretic

REPRODUCTIVE SYSTEM
- can be aphrodisiac especially sesquiterpenols

Alcohols are gentle but powerful in action. Some sesquiterpenols and aromatic alcohols may be calming.

■ Phenols and Phenolic Ethers

NERVOUS SYSTEM
- analgesic, antispasmodic, sedative stimulant, uplifting, warming

ENDOCRINE SYSTEM
- hormone like, stimulates secretions, reduces sweating, raises temperature

CIRCULATION AND IMMUNE SYSTEM
- antiviral, bactericidal, raises blood pressure, decongestant, stimulant especially for the immune system

SKIN, MUSCLE AND BODY TISSUES
- antiinflammatory, antiseptic, muscle toners, parasiticide, good for scar tissue

RESPIRATORY SYSTEM
- antiviral, bactericidal, expectorant, mucolytic

DIGESTIVE SYSTEM
- antiviral, bactericidal, decongestant, stimulant, vermifuge

URINARY SYSTEM
- diuretic, tonic

REPRODUCTIVE SYSTEM
- emmenagogue, stimulant

Phenols should be used with care particularly during pregnancy.

Introduction to Caddy Classic Profiles

For every batch of oil purchased a distributor is well advised to get a sample analysed to check its quality to make sure that it has not been adulterated. The most common way to do this is to send it to a laboratory for a Gas Liquid Chromatography (GC). The laboratory send the distributor a chromatograph of the oil. This is a graph that shows a series of peaks against a time scale. Each peak represents a chemical constituent that is present in the oil and the area of the peak gives the percentage of that constituent in the oil. Thus this graph can be compared with graphs of known pure oils to check its purity.

Harvest conditions, climate, extraction processes and storage conditions can all cause variations in the percentages of chemical constituents present in any batch of oils. However by considering the results of hundreds of batches of an oil together with historical data about its chemical make up it is possible to produce a classic profile giving acceptable ranges for the main constituents of an oil.

To create the ninety Caddy Classic Profiles that are given in Part 2 of this book an exhaustive search of the historical data on the make up of the oils listed and many GC's of batches of these oils have been collected. The percentages used to draw the Caddy Classic Profile for each oil are the averages of all these figures. The chemical constituents have been clustered into their chemical families to give the final data for the Caddy Classic Profiles.

Thus in Part 2 of this book you have a classic picture of each oil that communicates its nature.

The Caddy Classic Profile can also be used by anyone wishing to check whether their oils are of good quality and not adulterated.

At the foot of each page individual chemical constituents are listed and colour coded against their chemical families. The constituents that have been underlined are those most likely to be annotated on a chromatograph of the oil.

DILL (Anethum graveolens)

Caddy Classic Profile Colour visual - simple powerful picture.

Averaged ranges of chemical families in percentages.

ketones	50.0%
lactones and coumarins	3.0%
remainder	7.0%
monoterpenes	40.0%
phenols,phe.ethers	yes

Properties of oil, these apply to all body systems.

Stimulating   Balancing   Relaxing

PROPERTIES > USES

antispasmodic, sedative > crisis, headaches, shock

BODY SYSTEMS

NERVOUS SYSTEM

ENDOCRINE SYSTEM

increases sweating, stimulates milk production, stimulates secretions >

CIRCULATION AND IMMUNE SYSTEM

anticoagulant, bactericidal > arteries

SKIN, MUSCLES and BODY TISSUES

antifungal, antiseptic > wounds

Chemical families that best match uses for this body system.

RESPIRATORY SYSTEM

mucolytic > bronchitis, catarrh, fevers

DIGESTIVE SYSTEM

stimulates secretions > bile, flatulence, **indigestion**

Therapeutic uses of oil, in black, matched to most relevant body system.

URINARY SYSTEM

REPRODUCTIVE SYSTEM

stimulant > assists childbirth, stimulates milk production

CAUTIONS

Avoid in pregnancy. Use with care.

BOTANICAL FAMILY

Umbelliferae : This family generally aids digestion.

Botanical Family.

Herb: distilled Indian seeds : grasslike spicy aroma : top note. Historically used as a charm against witchcraft. Icelandic word dilla means soothing child. There are several different chemotypes.

Further information concerning the oil.

Chemical constituents may include:

carvone, dihydrocarvone, umbelliferone, umbelliprenin

limonene, phellandrene, cymene, terpinene

Individual chemical constituents.

Layout of information in Part 2 pages 1-90

1-16

2 | Caddy Classic Profiles

AMYRIS
Amyris balsamifera

■	esters	1.0%
■	aliphatic aldehydes	yes
■	sesquiterpenes	20.0%
□	lactones and coumarins	yes
▨	remainder	9.0%
■	alcohols	70.0%

Stimulating   Balancing   Relaxing

BODY SYSTEMS

NERVOUS SYSTEM
■ ■ ■ ■

ENDOCRINE SYSTEM
■

CIRCULATION AND IMMUNE SYSTEM
■ ■ ■ ■ ■

SKIN, MUSCLES AND BODY TISSUES
■ ■ ■ ■ ■

RESPIRATORY SYSTEM
■ ■ ■

DIGESTIVE SYSTEM
■ ■ ■ ■

URINARY SYSTEM
■ ■ ■

REPRODUCTIVE SYSTEM
■ ■ ■

PROPERTIES > USES

antispasmodic, calming >

warming >

antiviral, bactericidal, lowers blood pressure, decongestant > haemorrhoids, stimulates immune system, varicose veins

antiinflammatory, antiseptic > especially good for muscle cramps, rashes

bactericidal > bronchitis

calming > spasms

antiseptic > infections

antiseptic > infections

BOTANICAL FAMILY

Rutaceae : this family generally aids digestion and skin problems.

Tree: distilled wood and branches : musty wood aroma : base note.
Sometimes called West Indian Sandalwood or Rosewood which can lead to confusion. It grows in abundance in Haiti and is often called 'candlewood' as its twigs make excellent torches.

Chemical constituents may include:

■ caryophyllene, cadinene   □ furfural

■ amyrolin   ■ cadinol, balsamiol

1

BASIL EUGENOL
Ocimum gratissimum eugenoliferum

esters	0.6%
sesquiterpenes	12.0%
remainder	1.4%
monoterpenes	16.0%
alcohols	10.0%
phenols,phe. ethers	60.0%

Stimulating   Balancing   Relaxing

BODY SYSTEMS	PROPERTIES > USES
NERVOUS SYSTEM ■■■■■	calming, tonic > calms excitement
ENDOCRINE SYSTEM ■■■	hormone like > prostate
CIRCULATION AND IMMUNE SYSTEM ■■■■	antiviral, bactericidal >
SKIN, MUSCLES AND BODY TISSUES ■■■■■	antiseptic, parasiticide > arthritis, rheumatism
RESPIRATORY SYSTEM ■■■■■	decongestant, stimulant > bronchitis, pneumonia
DIGESTIVE SYSTEM ■■■	parasiticide, tonic > liver, pancreas, parasites
URINARY SYSTEM ■■■	decongestant > prostate
REPRODUCTIVE SYSTEM ■■■■	antiseptic > infections

CAUTIONS	Use with care because of the high phenol content.
BOTANICAL FAMILY	Lamiaceae.

Herb: distilled flowering herb : hearty warming aroma : top note.
Ocimum gratissimum eugenoliferum is a distinct oil from ocimum gratissimum thymoliferum with eugenol as its main phenol content. Maximum oil quantities are obtained during mass blooming time. The eugenol content drops by 10% two days after harvesting.

Chemical constituents may include:

■ cadinene   ■ α-terpineol, linalool

■ α-pinene, β-pinene, ocimene   ■ eugenol, methyl chavicol(estragole)

BASIL EXOTIC REUNION
Ocimum basilicum

■ esters	yes
■ ketones	1.0%
■ sesquiterpenes	yes
□ remainder	4.5%
□ oxides	2.5%
■ monoterpenes	yes
■ alcohols	2.0%
■ phenols,phe. ethers	90.0%

Stimulating   Balancing   Relaxing

BODY SYSTEMS	PROPERTIES > USES
NERVOUS SYSTEM ■ ■ ■ □ ■ ■	slightly antispasmodic > anxiety, balances sympathetic nervous system, depression
ENDOCRINE SYSTEM □ □ ■ ■	hormone like > prostate
CIRCULATION AND IMMUNE SYSTEM □ ■ □ ■ ■ ■	antiviral, slightly bactericidal, decongestant > pulmonary artery, yellow fever, veins
SKIN, MUSCLES AND BODY TISSUES ■ ■ □ ■ □ ■ ■ ■	antiinflammatory, antiseptic > plaques, polio, rheumatoid arthritis, tropical infections
RESPIRATORY SYSTEM ■ ■ ■ ■ ■	antiviral, slightly bactericidal > bronchitis, pneumonia
DIGESTIVE SYSTEM ■ ■ ■ □ ■ ■ ■	antiinflammatory > gastritis, liver, pancreas
URINARY SYSTEM □ □ ■ ■ ■	decongestant > prostate

REPRODUCTIVE SYSTEM

CAUTIONS

Use with care because of the high (85%) methyl chavicol content. Avoid in pregnancy.

BOTANICAL FAMILY
Lamiaceae.

Herb: distilled flowering herb : sweet herby with camphor tones aroma : top note. Although botanically classified the same as French or European Basil it is a larger plant with stronger odour and different constituents. Some practitioners discourage its use in aromatherapy.

Chemical constituents may include:

■ fenchyl acetate, linalyl acetate

□ α-pinene, β-pinene

□ octanone, camphor

■ terpinen-4-ol, α-terpineol, linalool, fenchol, citronellol

□ 1.8-cineole, *trans*-ocimene oxide

■ methyl chavicol(estragole), eugenol, *trans*-anethole, methyl eugenol

BASIL SWEET EUROPEAN
Ocimum basilicum

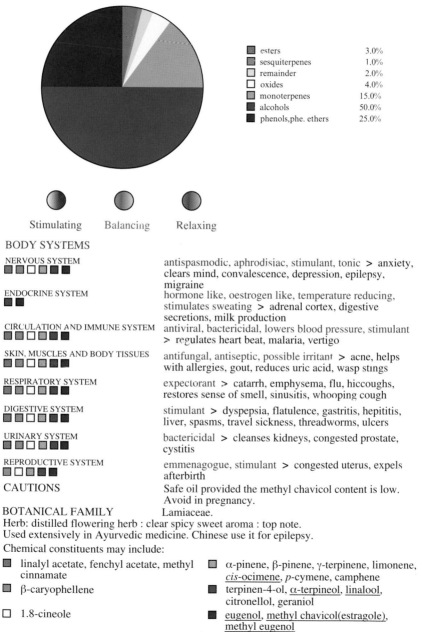

esters	3.0%
sesquiterpenes	1.0%
remainder	2.0%
oxides	4.0%
monoterpenes	15.0%
alcohols	50.0%
phenols,phe. ethers	25.0%

Stimulating Balancing Relaxing

BODY SYSTEMS

NERVOUS SYSTEM
■■□■■■
antispasmodic, aphrodisiac, stimulant, tonic > anxiety, clears mind, convalescence, depression, epilepsy, migraine

ENDOCRINE SYSTEM
■■
hormone like, oestrogen like, temperature reducing, stimulates sweating > adrenal cortex, digestive secretions, milk production

CIRCULATION AND IMMUNE SYSTEM
■■□■■■
antiviral, bactericidal, lowers blood pressure, stimulant > regulates heart beat, malaria, vertigo

SKIN, MUSCLES AND BODY TISSUES
■■□■■■
antifungal, antiseptic, possible irritant > acne, helps with allergies, gout, reduces uric acid, wasp stings

RESPIRATORY SYSTEM
■■□■■■
expectorant > catarrh, emphysema, flu, hiccoughs, restores sense of smell, sinusitis, whooping cough

DIGESTIVE SYSTEM
■■□■■■
stimulant > dyspepsia, flatulence, gastritis, hepititis, liver, spasms, travel sickness, threadworms, ulcers

URINARY SYSTEM
■■□■■■
bactericidal > cleanses kidneys, congested prostate, cystitis

REPRODUCTIVE SYSTEM
■□■■■
emmenagogue, stimulant > congested uterus, expels afterbirth

CAUTIONS
Safe oil provided the methyl chavicol content is low. Avoid in pregnancy.

BOTANICAL FAMILY
Lamiaceae.

Herb: distilled flowering herb : clear spicy sweet aroma : top note.
Used extensively in Ayurvedic medicine. Chinese use it for epilepsy.

Chemical constituents may include:

- ■ linalyl acetate, fenchyl acetate, methyl cinnamate
- ■ β-caryophellene
- □ 1.8-cineole

- ■ α-pinene, β-pinene, γ-terpinene, limonene, cis-ocimene, p-cymene, camphene
- ■ terpinen-4-ol, α-terpineol, linalool, citronellol, geraniol
- ■ eugenol, methyl chavicol(estragole), methyl eugenol

BASIL THYMOL
Ocimum gratissimum thymoliferum

■ sesquiterpenes	5.0%
☐ remainder	2.0%
☐ acids	yes
■ monoterpenes	38.0%
■ alcohols	5.0%
■ phenols,phe. ethers	50.0%

Stimulating   Balancing   Relaxing

BODY SYSTEMS	PROPERTIES > USES
NERVOUS SYSTEM ■■■	tonic >
ENDOCRINE SYSTEM	
CIRCULATION AND IMMUNE SYSTEM ■■■■	antiviral, bactericidal, stimulant > balances immune system
SKIN, MUSCLES AND BODY TISSUES ■■	antifungal, parasiticide >
RESPIRATORY SYSTEM ■■■■	bactericidal > bronchitis, pneumonia
DIGESTIVE SYSTEM ■■■	antiviral > enteritis
URINARY SYSTEM ■■■■	bactericidal > excellent for cystitis
REPRODUCTIVE SYSTEM	
CAUTIONS	Use with care. Avoid in pregnancy.
BOTANICAL FAMILY	Lamiaceae.

Herb: distilled flowering herb : herby warming aroma : top note.
Ocimum gratissimum thymoliferum is a distinct oil from ocimum gratissimum eugenoliferum with thymol as its main phenol content.

Chemical constituents may include:

■ β-caryophyllene, α-humulene, β-selinene

☐ α-thujene, α-pinene, β-pinene, myrcene, terpinenes, p-cymene

■ terpinen-4-ol, α-terpineol

■ thymol, carvacrol, eugenol, eugenol methyl ether, thymol methyl ether

BENZOIN
Styrax benzoin

■ esters		70.0%
☐ remainder		15.0%
☐ acids		15.0%
■ aromatic aldehydes		yes

Stimulating   Balancing   Relaxing

BODY SYSTEMS	PROPERTIES > USES
NERVOUS SYSTEM ■ ■	cheering, uplifting > comforting, clears mind, depression, loneliness, sadness
ENDOCRINE SYSTEM ■ ☐ ☐	stimulates secretions > balances blood sugar, pancreas
CIRCULATION AND IMMUNE SYSTEM ■ ☐ ☐ ■	astringent, tonic > cardiac, warms circulation
SKIN, MUSCLES AND BODY TISSUES ■ ☐ ■	antioxidant, antiseptic, deodorant > arthritis, dry cracked skin, eczema, itching, rheumatism, psoriasis, ulcers, wounds
RESPIRATORY SYSTEM ☐ ☐	expectorant, decongestant, mucolytic > catarrh
DIGESTIVE SYSTEM ■	calming > diabetes, flatulence
URINARY SYSTEM ☐ ☐ ■	diuretic > cystitis
REPRODUCTIVE SYSTEM ☐ ☐ ■	antiseptic, mucolytic > leucorrhoea

BOTANICAL FAMILY	Styracaceae.

Tree: gum solvent : vanilla like aroma : base note.
The sap is extracted and resin is solvent extracted - strictly speaking not an essential oil. It was used in ancient times to fend off evil spirits. Used in fumigations and in incense. It is an ingredient of Friar's Balsam.

Chemical constituents may include:

■ coniferyl benzoate, coniferyl cinnamate ■ benzaldehyde, vanillin

☐ benzoic acid, cinnamic acid

BERGAMOT
Citrus bergamia

■	esters	40.0%
■	aliphatic aldehydes	1.0%
■	sesquiterpenes	0.5%
■	lactones and coumarins	5.0%
□	remainder	2.5%
□	acids	yes
■	monoterpenes	33.0%
■	alcohols	18.0%

Stimulating   Balancing   Relaxing

BODY SYSTEMS

PROPERTIES > USES

NERVOUS SYSTEM
■ ■ ■

antispasmodic, calming > excellent for agitation, often first choice in cases of depression

ENDOCRINE SYSTEM
■

stimulates secretions > bile

CIRCULATION AND IMMUNE SYSTEM
■ ■ ■

antiviral, bactericidal >

SKIN, MUSCLES AND BODY TISSUES
■ ■ ■ ■ ■ ■

antifungal, antiseptic, phototoxic > boils, chicken pox, cold sores, herpes, pruritus, psoriasis, shingles

RESPIRATORY SYSTEM
■ ■ ■ ■ ■

antiviral > colds, flu, tonsillitis

DIGESTIVE SYSTEM
■ ■ □

stimulates secretions > gall stones, indigestion, internal parasites

URINARY SYSTEM
■ ■ ■ ■ ■

antiseptic > cystitis

REPRODUCTIVE SYSTEM
■ ■ ■ ■ ■

antifungal, antiseptic > leucorrhoea, thrush

CAUTIONS

Use with care skin may be photosensitive after application(1).

BOTANICAL FAMILY

Rutaceae : this family generally aids digestion and skin problems.

Tree: cold expression peel of nearly ripe fruit : light citrus aroma : top note.
Has gentle action covering a wide range of therapeutic uses. Used in Earl Grey tea.

Chemical constituents may include:

■ linalyl acetate

■ citral

■ β-bisabolene

■ bergaptene

■ β-pinene, γ-terpinene, α-terpinene, limonene

■ linalool, geraniol

BLACK PEPPER
Piper nigrum

■ aliphatic aldehydes	yes
☐ ketones	4.0%
■ sesquiterpenes	30.0%
☐ remainder	2.3%
☐ oxides	0.6%
☐ acids	yes
■ aromatic aldehydes	0.1%
■ monoterpenes	60.0%
■ alcohols	3.0%
■ phenols,phe. ethers	yes

Stimulating   Balancing   Relaxing

BODY SYSTEMS	PROPERTIES > USES
NERVOUS SYSTEM ☐■☐■■■■	analgesic, aphrodisiac, antispasmodic, tonic > neuralgia, Raynaud's disease
ENDOCRINE SYSTEM ■■	lowers fever, temperature control >
CIRCULATION AND IMMUNE SYSTEM ☐■☐■■■■	antiviral, bactericidal, decongestant, stimulant > anaemia, angina, cardiac
SKIN, MUSCLES AND BODY TISSUES ☐■☐☐■■■■	antiseptic > aches and pains, bruises, chilblains, rheumatism, rheumatoid arthritis, toothache, temporary paralysis
RESPIRATORY SYSTEM ☐■☐■■◣	expectorant, decongestant > bronchitis, catarrh
DIGESTIVE SYSTEM ☐■☐■■■	stimulant > constipation, flatulence, indigestion, liver, pancreas, reduces fat, tones colon muscles
URINARY SYSTEM ☐☐■■■	diuretic >
REPRODUCTIVE SYSTEM ☐■■■	stimulant > frigidity

CAUTIONS   Use with care too much may overstimulate the kidneys.

BOTANICAL FAMILY   Piperaceae.

Shrub: distilled fruits : sharp spicy aroma : middle note.
Used for over 4000 years in India particularly for urinary and liver disorders.

Chemical constituents may include:

- ☐ piperitone, dihydrocarvone
- ■ β-caryophyllene, bisabolene
- ☐ caryophyllene oxide, 1.8-cineole
- ▨ piperonal

- ☐ limonene, α-pinene, β-pinene, sabinene, terpinenes, phellandrene, myrcene, camphene, thujene
- ■ terpinen-4-ol, α-terpineol, linalool
- ■ myristicin, safrole

CADE
Juniperus oxycedrus

■	esters	yes
■	aliphatic aldehydes	1.0%
□	ketones	3.0%
■	sesquiterpenes	60.0%
□	remainder	5.3%
□	acids	0.7%
■	alcohols	30.0%
■	phenols,phe. ethers	yes

Stimulating   Balancing   Relaxing

BODY SYSTEMS

PROPERTIES > USES

NERVOUS SYSTEM
■ ■ □ □ ■

analgesic, calming > anxiety

ENDOCRINE SYSTEM

CIRCULATION AND IMMUNE SYSTEM

SKIN, MUSCLES AND BODY TISSUES
■ ■ □ ■ □ ■ ■

antiinflammatory, antiseptic, parasiticide, possible
irritant > cuts, dandruff, dermititis, eczema, spots

RESPIRATORY SYSTEM

DIGESTIVE SYSTEM
□ ■

parasiticide > worms

URINARY SYSTEM

REPRODUCTIVE SYSTEM

CAUTIONS

Use with care when treating inflammatory conditions or
allergic skin conditions.

BOTANICAL FAMILY

Cupressaceae : this family generally aids nervous
tension, rheumatism and cellulite.

Tree: distilled wood : leathery aroma : base note.
Used extensively in dermatological creams and ointments as well as in veterinary
medicine. Historically used for cutaneous and chronic skin problems.

Chemical constituents may include:

□ carvone

■ cadinol, pseudo-cedrol

■ β-caryophyllene, cadinene, cedrene

■ p-cresol, guaiacol

CARAWAY SEED
Carum carvi

ketones	54.0%	
sesquiterpenes	0.1%	
lactones and coumarins	yes	
remainder	1.8%	
acids	yes	
aromatic aldehydes	0.1%	
monoterpenes	40.0%	
alcohols	4.0%	

Stimulating   Balancing   Relaxing

BODY SYSTEMS

PROPERTIES > USES

NERVOUS SYSTEM
■ ■ ■

antispasmodic, tonic > anger, vertigo

ENDOCRINE SYSTEM
■ ■ ■

hormone like, tonic > stimulates milk production and bile production

CIRCULATION AND IMMUNE SYSTEM
■ ■ ■ ■ ■

stimulant, bactericidal > blood purifier, immune stimulant, possible aid for cancer(2)

SKIN, MUSCLES AND BODY TISSUES
■ ■ ■ ■ ■

antifungal, antiseptic > cell regenerator, scalp problems, toothache

RESPIRATORY SYSTEM
■ ■ ■ ■ ■

mucolytic > bronchitis, catarrh

DIGESTIVE SYSTEM
■ ■ ■ ■

stimulant > calms gastric and intestinal spasms, flatulence, indigestion, stimulates bile production

URINARY SYSTEM

REPRODUCTIVE SYSTEM
■

abortive > stimulates milk production

CAUTIONS

Avoid for pregnant women, babies and young children.

BOTANICAL FAMILY

Umbelliferae : this family generally aids digestion.

Herb: distilled fruits, dried ripe seed : peppery sharp yet sweet aroma : top note.
Used widely in cooking - it aids digestion. Also used in aperitifs.

Chemical constituents may include:

■ carvone, dihydrocarvone
■ caryophyllene
■ cuminaldehyde

■ limonene, phellandrene
■ cis-carveol, dihydrocarveol

CARROT SEED
Daucus carota

■ esters	3.0%
■ sesquiterpenes	16.0%
□ remainder	33.0%
□ acids	yes
■ monoterpenes	22.0%
■ alcohols	26.0%
■ phenols,phe. ethers	yes

Stimulating   Balancing   Relaxing

BODY SYSTEMS	PROPERTIES > USES
NERVOUS SYSTEM ■ ■ ■ ■ ■	calming, tonic > anxiety
ENDOCRINE SYSTEM ■ ■ ■ ■	hormone like, tonic to hormone production > regulates menstrual cycle, thyroid regulator
CIRCULATION AND IMMUNE SYSTEM ■ ■ ■ ■	bactericidal, decongestant, lowers blood pressure > anaemia, dilates blood vessels, immune stimulant
SKIN, MUSCLES AND BODY TISSUES ■ ■ □ ■ ■ ■	antiaging, antiseptic, cell regenerator > chilblains, eczema, gout, psoriasis, excellent for skin care, ulcers, wounds
RESPIRATORY SYSTEM ■ ■ ■ ■	bactericidal > bronchitis, strengthens mucous membranes
DIGESTIVE SYSTEM ■ ■ ■ ■ ■	bactericidal, calming > anorexia, diarrhoea, flatulance, hepatitis, jaundice, liver problems, ulcers
URINARY SYSTEM ■ ■ ■ ■	diuretic > cystitis, purifies kidneys, kidney stones
REPRODUCTIVE SYSTEM ■ ■ ■ ■ ■	hormone like > aids conception, helps infertility

BOTANICAL FAMILY   Umbelliferae : this family generally aids digestion.

Plant wild carrot: distilled seed : dry sweet aroma : middle note.
Excellent for general health and well being. Used widely in food flavouring.

Chemical constituents may include:

■ geranyl acetate   ■ carotol, daucol, linalool, geraniol

■ daucene, bisabolene, elemene,   ■ asarone
  caryophyllene

■ limonene, α-pinene, β-pinene

11

CATNIP
Nepata cataria

esters		yes
aliphatic aldehydes		10.5%
sesquiterpenes		8.0%
lactones and coumarins		15.0%
remainder		2.5%
acids		yes
monoterpenes		2.0%
alcohols		62.0%
phenols,phe. ethers		yes

Stimulating   Balancing   Relaxing

BODY SYSTEMS	PROPERTIES > USES
NERVOUS SYSTEM ■■■■■	antispamodic, calming, uplifting > nervous depression
ENDOCRINE SYSTEM	
CIRCULATION AND IMMUNE SYSTEM ■□■■	strongly antiviral >
SKIN, MUSCLES AND BODY TISSUES ■■■■□□■■	antiinflammatory, antiseptic > arthritis, herpes, rheumatism
RESPIRATORY SYSTEM	
DIGESTIVE SYSTEM ■■■■■■	calming > gall stones, irritable bowel syndrome
URINARY SYSTEM ■■□■■	antiseptic > infections
REPRODUCTIVE SYSTEM	

BOTANICAL FAMILY   Lamiaceae.

Herb: distilled flower tips : strong pungent aroma due to nepetalactone : top note.
Unusual essential oil in its 15% lactones This ties up with its recommendation for nervous depression.

Chemical constituents may include:

■ neral, geranial

■ β-caryophyllene, α-humulene

□ nepetalactone, epinepetalactone, dihydronepetalactone

□ myrcene, limonene, ocimene

■ citronellol, geraniol

CEDAR TEXAS
Juniperus ashei

■	sesquiterpenes	60.0%
□	remainder	5.0%
■	alcohols	35.0%

Stimulating   Balancing   Relaxing

BODY SYSTEMS	PROPERTIES > USES
NERVOUS SYSTEM □ ■	antispasmodic, sedative > nervous tension, stress
ENDOCRINE SYSTEM	
CIRCULATION AND IMMUNE SYSTEM □ ■	astringent, bactericidal, decongestant, stimulant > phlebitis
SKIN, MUSCLES AND BODY TISSUES □ ■	antiseptic > acne, arthritis, dandruff, eczema, greasy hair, haemorrhoids, psoriasis, rheumatism, varicose veins
RESPIRATORY SYSTEM ■ □ ■	expectorant > bronchitis, catarrh, coughs, sinusitis
DIGESTIVE SYSTEM	
URINARY SYSTEM □ ■	diuretic > cystitis
REPRODUCTIVE SYSTEM □ ■	antiseptic > leucorrhoea
CAUTIONS	Can irritate skin. Avoid in pregnancy.
BOTANICAL FAMILY	Cupressaceae : this family generally aids nervous tension, rheumatism and cellulite.

Tree: distilled heartwood : sweet tar like aroma : base note.
Small 24 foot tree with crooked and twisted branches. It is felled for its essential oil.
Traditionally used to treat skin rashes, arthritis and rheumatism.

Chemical constituents may include:

□   cedrene, thujopsene   ■   cedrol, widdrol

CEDAR VIRGINIAN RED
Juniperus virginiana

▦ sesquiterpenes	60.0%
☐ remainder	10.0%
▪ alcohols	30.0%

Stimulating   Balancing   Relaxing

BODY SYSTEMS	PROPERTIES > USES
NERVOUS SYSTEM ▪▪	antispasmodic, good for meditation, sedative, tonic > nervous tension
ENDOCRINE SYSTEM ▪▪	balancing > controls sebum production, good for chronic conditions
CIRCULATION AND IMMUNE SYSTEM ▪▪	astringent, decongestant > internal and external haemorrhoids, phlebitis, ulcers
SKIN, MUSCLES AND BODY TISSUES ▪☐▪	antifungal, antiseptic, balm, insecticide > acne, baldness, chronic arthritis and rheumatism, dandruff, eczema, oily skin
RESPIRATORY SYSTEM ▪☐▪	expectorant > catarrh (drying effect), bronchitis
DIGESTIVE SYSTEM	
URINARY SYSTEM ▪▪	diuretic > cystitis (calms burning pain), kidney tonic
REPRODUCTIVE SYSTEM ☐▪	possibly abortive > leucorrhoea
CAUTIONS	Can irritate skin. Avoid in pregnancy.
BOTANICAL FAMILY	Cupressaceae : this family generally aids nervous tension, rheumatism and cellulite.

Tree: distilled sawdust, previously heartwood : dry sandalwood like aroma : base note. Large redwood 100 feet, trunk diameter 5 feet. Derivation of the word cedar means spiritual strength, symbol of good faith. Used as incense and in mummification.

Chemical constituents may include:

▦ cadinene, cedrene, thujopsene, cuparene ▪ cedrol, cedrenol, widdrol, γ-eudesmol

CEDARWOOD ATLAS
Cedrus atlantica

☐ ketones	19.0%
■ sesquiterpenes	50.0%
☐ remainder	2.0%
■ alcohols	29.0%

Stimulating   Balancing   Relaxing

BODY SYSTEMS	PROPERTIES > USES
NERVOUS SYSTEM ☐■■	aphrodisiac, sedative > neuralgia
ENDOCRINE SYSTEM ☐■■	balancing > balances sebum production
CIRCULATION AND IMMUNE SYSTEM ☐■■	bactericidal, decongestant > clears arteries, cellulite, stimulates lympth circulation
SKIN, MUSCLES AND BODY TISSUES ☐■■	antifungal, antiseptic > arthritis, hair loss, pruritus, rheumatism, wounds
RESPIRATORY SYSTEM ☐■■	mucolytic > bronchitis, TB
DIGESTIVE SYSTEM	
URINARY SYSTEM ☐■■	diuretic > cystitis
REPRODUCTIVE SYSTEM ☐	mucolytic > leucorrhoea
CAUTIONS	Best avoided in pregnancy.
BOTANICAL FAMILY	Pinaceae : this family is highly antiseptic and generally aids respiratory problems.

Tree: distilled wood : woody dry aroma : base note.
Majestic 120 foot tree . Hardwood with strong aroma. Traditionally used for bronchial and urinary tract infections also for preservation and incense. Employed in traditional Tibetan medicine.
Chemical constituents may include:

☐ α-atlantone, γ-atlantone   ■ atlantol, cedrol

■ cedrene, caryophyllene, thujopsene, cadinene

15

CHAMOMILE GERMAN
Matricaria recutica

■ sesquiterpenes		35.0%
■ lactones and coumarins		yes
□ remainder		9.0%
□ oxides		35.0%
■ monoterpenes		1.0%
■ alcohols		20.0%

Stimulating   Balancing   Relaxing

BODY SYSTEMS

NERVOUS SYSTEM
■ □ ■ ■ ■

ENDOCRINE SYSTEM
■ ■ □ ■ ■

CIRCULATION AND IMMUNE SYSTEM
■ ■ □ □ ■

SKIN, MUSCLES AND BODY TISSUES
■ ■ □ □ ■ ■

RESPIRATORY SYSTEM

DIGESTIVE SYSTEM
■ ■ ■ □ □ ■

URINARY SYSTEM
■ □ ■

REPRODUCTIVE SYSTEM
■ □ □ ■ ■

BOTANICAL FAMILY

PROPERTIES > USES

analgesic, antispasmodic(3) > insomnia, migraine, stress

hormone like, temperature reducing, stimulates secretions > balances menstrual cycle, bile

bactericidal, decongestant > fever, stimulates production of leucocytes

antiinflammatory > acne, allergies, boils, burns, insect bites, psoriasis, rashes, rheumatism, toothache, ulcers, wounds

calming, tonic, vermifuge > calms digestion, gastric ulcers, stimulates bile production

bactericidal > cystitis

balancing > amenorrhoea, heavy periods, painful periods

Compositae : this family is generally soothing especially for skin and digestion.

Herb: distilled flower heads : warm herby aroma : middle note.
Used in traditional medicine(4) good for all states of tension and nervous reactions to stress. The deep blue colour of the oil is due to the chamazulene which forms during distillation.

Chemical constituents may include:

■ chamazulene, farnesene

■ α-bisabolol(5)

□ α-bisabolol oxide

□ en-yn-dicycloether, *cis*-spiro ether

CHAMOMILE MAROC
Ormenis multicaulis

■	esters	3.5%
■	ketones	0.5%
■	sesquiterpenes	9.7%
☐	remainder	21.3%
☐	oxides	yes
■	monoterpenes	24.0%
■	alcohols	41.0%
■	phenols	yes

Stimulating   Balancing   Relaxing

BODY SYSTEMS

NERVOUS SYSTEM
■ ■ ■ ☐ ■ ■ ■

ENDOCRINE SYSTEM
☐ ■ ■ ■

CIRCULATION AND IMMUNE SYSTEM
■ ■ ☐ ■ ■ ■

SKIN, MUSCLES AND BODY TISSUES
■ ■ ■ ■ ■ ■

RESPIRATORY SYSTEM

DIGESTIVE SYSTEM
☐ ☐ ■ ■ ■

URINARY SYSTEM
■ ■ ☐ ■ ■

REPRODUCTIVE SYSTEM
■ ■ ■ ☐ ■ ■ ■

PROPERTIES > USES

aphrodisiac, tonic > depression, insomnia, irritability, headache

hormone like, stimulates secretions >

bactericidal, decongestant, general tonic > decongestant for arteries

antiseptic, parasiticide > eczema, dry cracked skin, infected pus

stimulates secretions > bile and gastric juices, liver and spleen congestion, parasites

bactericidal > cystitis, prostate problems

emmenagogue > amenorrhoea, menopause, painful periods

BOTANICAL FAMILY

Compositae : this family is generally soothing especially for the skin and digestion.

Herb: distilled flowerheads : fresh balsamic aroma : middle note.
Distantly related to the roman and german chamomiles.
Chemical constituents may include:

- ■ benzyl acetate, bornyl acetate, bornyl butyrate
- ☐ camphor, pinocarvone
- ■ germacrene, β-caryophyllene, bisabolene
- ☐ 1.8-cineole
- ■ α-pinene, myrcene
- ■ santolina alcohol, yomogi alcohol, artemisia alcohol, trans-pinocarveol
- ■ eugenol

17

CHAMOMILE ROMAN
Chamaemelum nobile

■	esters	75.0%
■	aliphatic aldehydes	2.0%
☐	ketones	3.0%
■	sesquiterpenes	3.0%
■	lactones and coumarins	yes
☐	remainder	2.0%
☐	oxides	5.0%
☐	acids	yes
■	monoterpenes	5.0%
■	alcohols	5.0%

Stimulating   Balancing   Relaxing

BODY SYSTEMS	PROPERTIES > USES
NERVOUS SYSTEM ■ ■ ■ ■ ■ ■	antispasmodic, calming, sedative > depression, insomnia, irritability, neuralgia, neuritis, migraine, shocks
ENDOCRINE SYSTEM ■ ■ ■ ■ ■	temperature reducing, causes sweating > balances menstrual cycle
CIRCULATION AND IMMUNE SYSTEM ☐ ☐ ■	bactericidal > anaemia
SKIN, MUSCLES AND BODY TISSUES ■ ■ ■ ■ ■ ☐ ☐ ■	antiinflammatory > back pain, conjunctivitis, cracked nipples, gout, irritation, psoriasis, surgical scars
RESPIRATORY SYSTEM ■ ■ ■ ■	calming > nervous asthma
DIGESTIVE SYSTEM ■ ■ ■ ■ ■ ☐ ■ ■	calming, parasiticide > intestinal colic, flatulence, jaundice, liver, stimulates appetite
URINARY SYSTEM	
REPRODUCTIVE SYSTEM ■ ■ ■ ■ ■ ☐ ■ ■	emmenagogue > amenorrhoea, nervous menstrual problems, menopause, painful periods
BOTANICAL FAMILY	Compositae : this family is soothing especially for the skin and digestion.

Herb: distilled flowerheads : fruity apple like aroma : middle note.
Highly respected for its calming influence on all systems. Known as the plant's physician as it protects neighbouring plants from infections. Potent sedative as well as long lasting antiinflammatory(6).

Chemical constituents may include:

■ angelates, tiglates, butyrates, propionates
☐ pinocarvone
■ chamazulene, caryophyllene

☐ 1.8-cineole
■ α-pinene, sabinene
■ farnesol, nerolidol, α-terpineol, *trans*-pinocarveol

CINNAMON LEAF
Cinnamomum zeylanicum

■ esters	yes
■ sesquiterpenes	4.0%
□ remainder	3.0%
■ aromatic aldehydes	5.0%
□ monoterpenes	yes
■ alcohols	2.0%
■ phenols,phe. ethers	86.0%

Stimulating   Balancing   Relaxing

BODY SYSTEMS

NERVOUS SYSTEM
■ ■ ■ ■ ■ ■

ENDOCRINE SYSTEM
■ ■ ■ ■

CIRCULATION AND IMMUNE SYSTEM
■ ■ ■ ■ ■ ■

SKIN, MUSCLES AND BODY TISSUES
■ ■ ■ ■ ■ ■

RESPIRATORY SYSTEM
■ ■ ■ ■ ■ ■

DIGESTIVE SYSTEM
■ ■ ■ ■ ■ ■

URINARY SYSTEM

REPRODUCTIVE SYSTEM
■

CAUTIONS

BOTANICAL FAMILY

PROPERTIES > USES

antispasmodic, aphrodisiac, stimulant > neuralgia

raises body temperature, stimulates secretions > gastric, glandular tonic, promotes menstruation, stimulates tears and mucous

antiviral, astringent, bactericidal, heart tonic > arrests bleeding, blood purifier

antifungal, antioxidant, antiseptic, tonic > insects, toothache, warts

antispasmodic > eases breathing, fainting fits

stimulates secretions > anorexia, diarrhoea, flatulence, nausea, saliva flow

emmenagogue > can help in childbirth, leucorrhoea

Avoid in pregnancy. Powerful oil use with care.

Lauraceae : this family is usually powerful and stimulating.

Tree: distilled leaves : musty sweet sharp aroma : base note.
Pheonix collected cinnamon, myrrh and spikenard for the magic fire. Cinnamon was used in love potions and incense.

Chemical constituents may include:

■ benzyl benzoate, benzyl acetate, cinnamyl acetate
■ β-caryophyllene
■ cinnamaldehyde, methyl vanillin

□ α-pinene, p-cymene

■ geraniol, borneol, linalool, terpineol

■ eugenol, safrole, aceteugenol

CLARY SAGE
Salvia sclarea

■ esters	70.0%
■ aliphatic aldehydes	yes
□ ketones	yes
■ sesquiterpenes	4.0%
■ lactones and coumarins	yes
□ remainder	3.2%
□ oxides	0.8%
□ acids	yes
■ monoterpenes	2.0%
■ alcohols	20.0%
■ phenols,phe. ethers	yes

Stimulating   Balancing   Relaxing

BODY SYSTEMS

PROPERTIES > USES

NERVOUS SYSTEM
■ ■ ■ ■ ■ □ ■ ■ ■

antispasmodic, calming, sedative, tonic > convalescence, convulsions, panic attacks, postnatal depression

ENDOCRINE SYSTEM
□ ■ ■ ■

controls sebum production, oestrogen like, stops sweating > menopausal problems

CIRCULATION AND IMMUNE SYSTEM
■ ■ ■ ■ □ ■ ■ ■

slightly bactericidal, decongestant, lowers blood pressure > cholesterol, phlebitis, varicose veins

SKIN, MUSCLES AND BODY TISSUES
■ ■ ■ ■ ■ ■ ■

antifungal, antiinflammatory, deodorant > baldness, dandruff, greasy hair, haemorrhoids , mature skin, puffy skin

RESPIRATORY SYSTEM
■ ■ ■ ■ ■

calming > asthma

DIGESTIVE SYSTEM
■ ■ ■ ■ ■ □ ■

calming > diabetes, flatulence

URINARY SYSTEM

REPRODUCTIVE SYSTEM
■ ■ ■ ■ ■ □ ■ ■ ■

uterine tonic > amenorrhoea, assists childbirth, menopausal problems, scanty periods

CAUTIONS

Avoid in cases of hormone related cancers. Avoid in pregnancy. Do not use if alcohol has been consumed.

BOTANICAL FAMILY

Lamiaceae.

Herb: distilled flower stalks : nutty earthy aroma : top note.
Name comes from 'clarus' meaning clear and was used for clearing mucous from the eyes. There are several different chemotypes, some oils are lower in esters and higher in alcohols.

Chemical constituents may include:

■ linalyl acetate, geranyl acetate, neryl acetate
■ caryophyllenal
□ thujone, camphor
■ caryophyllene, germacrene, bourbonene

□ 1.8-cineole, caryophyllene oxide
■ α-pinene, β-pinene, myrcene, limonene, phellandrene
■ linalool, sclareol, α-terpineol, α-bisabolol
■ methyl hexyl ether

CLOVE BUD
Syzygium aromaticum

■ esters	yes
■ sesquiterpenes	6.0%
□ remainder	3.0%
□ oxides	1.0%
■ monoterpenes	yes
■ phenols,phe. ethers	90.0%

Stimulating   Balancing   Relaxing

BODY SYSTEMS	PROPERTIES > USES
NERVOUS SYSTEM ■ ■ □ ■ ■	analgesic, antispasmodic, stimulating > memory loss, neuralgia, polio, Raynaud's disease
ENDOCRINE SYSTEM □ ■ ■	hormone like > balances thyroid problems
CIRCULATION AND IMMUNE SYSTEM □ ■ ■	antiviral, bactericidal, raises blood pressure > chlorosis, Hodgkin's disease
SKIN, MUSCLES AND BODY TISSUES ■ ■ □ ■ ■	antioxidant , strong air antiseptic > clothes moths, herpes, infected acne, mosquitoes, rheumatoid arthritis, toothache, ulcers, wounds
RESPIRATORY SYSTEM ■ □ ■ ■	bactericidal > bronchitis, sinusitis, TB
DIGESTIVE SYSTEM ■ ■ ■ ■	stimulates secretions > bowel spasm, dysentery, enteritis, liver tonic, saliva
URINARY SYSTEM ■ ■ □ ■ ■	tonic > cystitis, kidney tonic
REPRODUCTIVE SYSTEM ■ ■ ■ ■	uterine tonic > assists childbirth, frigidity, impotence, muscle toner
CAUTIONS	Check for skin irritation. Use well diluted < 1%.
BOTANICAL FAMILY	Myrtaceae : this family is generally stimulating and good for the respiratory tract.

Tree: distilled buds : strong spicy aroma : base note.
Used in traditional medicine for alleviating toothache. It prevents the spread of contagious diseases such as plague. Used in many modern pharmaceuticals.

Chemical constituents may include:

■ β-caryophyllene, humulenes	■ pinenes
□ caryophyllene oxide, humulene oxide	■ eugenol, isoeugenol, aceteugenol

CORIANDER
Coriandrum sativum

■ esters	3.0%
▨ aliphatic aldehydes	yes
☐ ketones	8.0%
■ lactones and coumarins	yes
☐ remainder	4.0%
☐ acids	yes
■ monoterpenes	15.0%
■ alcohols	70.0%
■ phenols,phe. ethers	yes

Stimulating   Balancing   Relaxing

BODY SYSTEMS	PROPERTIES > USES
NERVOUS SYSTEM ■■■■■■	analgesic, antispasmodic, euphoric, uplifting, tonic > mental fatigue, sadness
ENDOCRINE SYSTEM ■■	hormone like, stimulates secretions > balances menstrual cycle, glandular tonic, warming
CIRCULATION AND IMMUNE SYSTEM ■■■■■■	anticoagulant, antiviral, bactericidal > purifies system
SKIN, MUSCLES AND BODY TISSUES ■■■■■■■	antiseptic, parasiticide > osteoarthritis, rheumatism
RESPIRATORY SYSTEM ■■■■	antiviral > flu, lungs
DIGESTIVE SYSTEM ■■■■■■■	tonic > anorexia, colic, bad breath, enteritis, indigestion
URINARY SYSTEM ■■■■■	bactericidal > cystitis
REPRODUCTIVE SYSTEM ■■■■	stimulates secretions > irregular periods, vaginal

BOTANICAL FAMILY   Umbelliferae : this family generally aids digestion.

Herb: distilled seeds : sweet spicy woody aroma : top note.
Used since ancient times considered the herb of happiness with aphrodisiac properties. It is used in Benedictene and Chatreuse liqueurs.

Chemical constituents may include:

- ■ geranyl acetate, linalyl acetate
- ■ decyl aldehyde
- ☐ camphor, carvone
- ☐ umbelliferone, bergaptene

- ☐ γ-terpinene, p-cymene, α-pinene, limonene
- ■ linalool, α-terpineol, geraniol, borneol
- ■ anethole

CYPRESS
Cupressus sempervirens

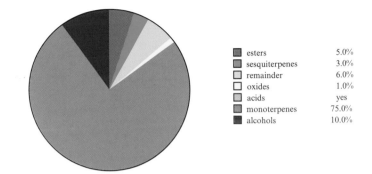

■ esters	5.0%
■ sesquiterpenes	3.0%
□ remainder	6.0%
□ oxides	1.0%
■ acids	yes
■ monoterpenes	75.0%
■ alcohols	10.0%

Stimulating   Balancing   Relaxing

BODY SYSTEMS	PROPERTIES > USES
NERVOUS SYSTEM ■■□■■	antispasmodic, balances sympathetic nerve system, tonic > irritability
ENDOCRINE SYSTEM ■■■■	balancing, reduces sweating > regulates ovarian function, combats excesses
CIRCULATION AND IMMUNE SYSTEM ■■□■■	astringent, bactericidal, decongestant > constricts blood vessels
SKIN, MUSCLES AND BODY TISSUES ■■■□■■■	antiseptic, insecticide > broken capillaries , cellulite, haemorrhoids, pyorrhoea, rheumatism, sweaty feet
RESPIRATORY SYSTEM ■■■□■■■	bactericidal > bronchitis, lungs, pleurisy, TB, whooping cough
DIGESTIVE SYSTEM □■.■	stimulates secretions > liver, pancreas
URINARY SYSTEM □■■	decongestant, diuretic > prostate problems
REPRODUCTIVE SYSTEM ■■■	balancing > irregular periods, menopause, pmt
BOTANICAL FAMILY	Cupressaceae : this family generally aids nervous tension, rheumatism and cellulite.

Tree: distilled needles and twigs : clear woody spicy aroma : base note.
The island of Cypress was named after this tree. The tree was worshipped and statues of the gods carved out of it. Sempervirens means lives for ever.

Chemical constituents may include:

■ α-terpinyl acetate, terpinen-4-yl acetate   □ α-pinene, β-pinene, Δ^3-carene , p-cymene, camphene, limonene

■ cedrene, cadinene   ■ cedrol, α-terpineol, borneol, sabinol, manool

□ 1.8-cineole, manoyl oxide

DILL
Anethum graveolens

ketones	50.0%
lactones and coumarins	3.0%
remainder	7.0%
monoterpenes	40.0%
phenols,phe.ethers	yes

Stimulating   Balancing   Relaxing

BODY SYSTEMS	PROPERTIES > USES
NERVOUS SYSTEM	antispasmodic, sedative > crisis, headaches, shock
ENDOCRINE SYSTEM	increases sweating, stimulates milk production, stimulates secretions >
CIRCULATION AND IMMUNE SYSTEM	anticoagulant, bactericidal > arteries
SKIN, MUSCLES AND BODY TISSUES	antifungal, antiseptic > wounds
RESPIRATORY SYSTEM	mucolytic > bronchitis, catarrh, fevers
DIGESTIVE SYSTEM	stimulates secretions > bile, flatulence, indigestion
URINARY SYSTEM	
REPRODUCTIVE SYSTEM	stimulant > assists childbirth, stimulates milk production

CAUTIONS   Avoid in pregnancy. Use with care.

BOTANICAL FAMILY   Umbelliferae : This family generally aids digestion.

Herb: distilled Indian seeds : grasslike spicy aroma : top note.
Historically used as a charm against witchcraft. Icelandic word dilla means soothing child.
There are several different chemotypes.

Chemical constituents may include:

carvone, dihydrocarvone

umbelliferone, umbelliprenin

limonene, phellandrene, cymene, terpinene

EUCALYPTUS BLUE GUM
Eucalyptus globulus

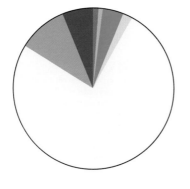

▪	esters	1.0%
▪	aliphatic aldehydes	yes
▫	ketones	1.0%
▪	sesquiterpenes	4.0%
▫	remainder	2.0%
▫	oxides	76.0%
▫	acids	yes
▪	monoterpenes	10.0%
▪	alcohols	6.0%

Stimulating   Balancing   Relaxing

BODY SYSTEMS	PROPERTIES > USES
NERVOUS SYSTEM ■■□■□■	stimulant > clears head, cools emotions, migraine
ENDOCRINE SYSTEM ■■□■	stimulates secretions, temperature reducing > colds, lowers blood sugar, gall bladder, pancreas
CIRCULATION AND IMMUNE SYSTEM ■■□■□■	antiviral, decongestant > malaria, reduces haemorrhage, typhoid
SKIN, MUSCLES AND BODY TISSUES ■■■■□■■■	antiseptic > arthritis, athlete's foot, chicken pox, gnats, herpes, measles, mosquitoes
RESPIRATORY SYSTEM ■■■■□■■■	decongestant, expectorant, mucolytic > asthma, catarrh, diphtheria, laryngitis, pneumonia, scarlet fever, tonsillitis
DIGESTIVE SYSTEM □□■	stimulates secretions > diabetes, gall stones, pancreas
URINARY SYSTEM ■■□■■	antiseptic > cystitis, nephritis
REPRODUCTIVE SYSTEM ■■□□■	antiseptic > candida, gonorrhoea, leucorrhoea

BOTANICAL FAMILY	Myrtaceae : This family is generally stimulating and good for the respiratory system.

Tree: distilled leaves and twigs : harsh camphor like aroma : top note.
An excellent oil for coughs, colds and flu.

Chemical constituents may include:

- ■ α-terpinyl acetate
- ▫ pinocarvone
- ■ aromadendrene

- □ 1.8-cineole, α-pinene epoxide
- ▪ α-pinene, limonene, *p-cymene*, phellandrene
- ▪ globulol, *trans*-pinocarveol

EUCALYPTUS DIVES
Eucalyptus dives

■ aliphatic aldehydes	yes
□ ketones	45.0%
■ sesquiterpenes	yes
□ remainder	21.0%
□ acids	yes
■ monoterpenes	30.0%
■ alcohols	4.0%

Stimulating   Balancing   Relaxing

BODY SYSTEMS   PROPERTIES > USES

NERVOUS SYSTEM   calming, sedative > exhaustion, headaches, nervous
■ ■ ■ ■   sciatica, neuralgia

ENDOCRINE SYSTEM   temperature reducing >
■ □

CIRCULATION AND IMMUNE SYSTEM   anticoagulant >
□

SKIN, MUSCLES AND BODY TISSUES antiseptic > arthritis, cuts, rheumatism, sores, ulcers
■ □ □ □ ■

RESPIRATORY SYSTEM   expectorant, decongestant, mucolytic > asthma,
■ □ □ □ ■   bronchitis, catarrh, sinusitis

DIGESTIVE SYSTEM   stimulates secretions > gastric, aids liver function
□ □

URINARY SYSTEM   diuretic > kidney diseases, kidney tonic
□ □ ■

REPRODUCTIVE SYSTEM   abortive > leucorrhoea
□

CAUTIONS   Avoid in pregnancy and babies and young children.

BOTANICAL FAMILY   Myrtaceae : this family is generally stimulating and
                             good for the respiratory system.

Tree: distilled leaves and twigs : camphor like spicy minty aroma : top note.
Aborigines burnt the leaves believing that the heat left the sick man and went into the fire.

Chemical constituents may include:

□ piperitone   □ α-phellandrene, camphene, p-cymene,
                               terpinene, thujene

■ β-caryophyllene   ■ terpinen-4-ol, α-terpineol, linalool,
                               piperitol

EUCALYPTUS LEMON SCENTED
Eucalyptus citriodora

esters	3.0%	
aliphatic aldehydes	80.0%	
ketones	yes	
remainder	4.0%	
oxides	1.0%	
monoterpenes	yes	
alcohols	12.0%	

Stimulating   Balancing   Relaxing

BODY SYSTEMS

NERVOUS SYSTEM

ENDOCRINE SYSTEM

CIRCULATION AND IMMUNE SYSTEM

SKIN, MUSCLES AND BODY TISSUES

RESPIRATORY SYSTEM

DIGESTIVE SYSTEM

URINARY SYSTEM

REPRODUCTIVE SYSTEM

BOTANICAL FAMILY

PROPERTIES > USES

antispasmodic, calming >

antiviral, bactericidal, lowers blood pressure > coronary, fever

antifungal, antiinflammatory, antiseptic > arthritis, chicken pox, dandruff, herpes, insects, rheumatism, scabs, sores, wounds

calming > allergies, asthma, laryngitis, sore throat

antiseptic > cystitis

stimulates secretions > excellent for candida, vaginal

Myrtaceae : this family is generally stimulating and good for the respiratory system.

Tree: distilled leaves and twigs : lemon tinged aroma : top note.
Due to its pleasant aroma it was used to perfume linen stores and to protect against silverfish and cockroaches. The synergistic action of this oil has been shown to be four times that of its components(7).

Chemical constituents may include:

- citronellyl butyrate, citronellyl citronellate, citronellyl acetate
- citronellal
- menthone

- 1.8-cineole
- α-pinene
- citronellol, geraniol, *trans*-pinocarveol

EUCALYPTUS SMITHII
Eucalyptus smithii

▨	esters	yes
◧	aliphatic aldehydes	1.0%
◨	sesquiterpenes	1.0%
☐	remainder	2.0%
☐	oxides	78.0%
▨	monoterpenes	17.0%
■	alcohols	1.0%
■	phenols,phe. ethers	yes

Stimulating   Balancing   Relaxing

BODY SYSTEMS

NERVOUS SYSTEM
■ ■ ■ ☐ ■ ■ ■

ENDOCRINE SYSTEM

CIRCULATION AND IMMUNE SYSTEM
■ ■ ■ ■

SKIN, MUSCLES AND BODY TISSUES
■ ■ ■ ☐ ■ ■ ■

RESPIRATORY SYSTEM
■ ☐ ■ ■ ■

DIGESTIVE SYSTEM
☐ ■ ■ ■

URINARY SYSTEM

REPRODUCTIVE SYSTEM

PROPERTIES > USES

analgesic, calming(evening), stimulating(morning) > headaches

antiviral > colds, flu

antiseptic > painful joints and muscles

decongestant > asthma, bronchitis, catarrh, coughs

stimulant >

BOTANICAL FAMILY   Myrtaceae : this family is generally stimulating and good for the respiratory system.

Tree: distilled leaves and twigs : penetrating aroma : top note.
Extremely high proportion of oxide gives it similar properties to eucalyptus globulus.

Chemical constituents may include:

■   isovaleraldehyde   ☐   1.8-cineole

◧   limonene, α-pinene, p-cymene   ■   terpineol, geraniol, linalool, eudesmol

EUCALYPTUS STAIGERIANA
Eucalyptus staigeriana

esters		8.6%
aliphatic aldehydes		21.3%
ketones		5.6%
sesquiterpenes		2.5%
remainder		16.2%
oxides		5.0%
monoterpenes		34.5%
alcohols		6.3%

Stimulating   Balancing   Relaxing

BODY SYSTEMS

NERVOUS SYSTEM
■ ■ □ ■ □

ENDOCRINE SYSTEM

CIRCULATION AND IMMUNE SYSTEM
□ □ ■ ■

SKIN, MUSCLES AND BODY TISSUES
■ ■ □ ■ ■ ■

RESPIRATORY SYSTEM
■ □ ■ □ ■ ■

DIGESTIVE SYSTEM
■ ■ □ ■

URINARY SYSTEM

REPRODUCTIVE SYSTEM
□ ■ ■

BOTANICAL FAMILY

PROPERTIES > USES

analgesic, calming > relaxes solar plexus

decongestant, stimulant >

antiinflammatory, antiseptic > backpain, bites, rashes, neckache, muscle cramps, sores, stings, wounds

gentle decongestant > sinusitis, sore throat

calming > digestive spasms

sexual tonic >

Myrtaceae : this family is generally stimulating and good for the respiratory system.

Tree: distilled leaves and twigs : light lemon aroma : top note.
It is likely that this eucalyptus oil is gentler than most other eucalyptus oils and might be considered for use with the elderly or young.

Chemical constituents may include:

■ menthyl acetate, geranyl acetate   ■ limonene, *p*-cymene

■ neral, geranial   ■ nerol, geraniol

FENNEL SWEET
Foeniculum vulgare

☐ ketones	5.0%
☐ lactones and coumarins	yes
☐ remainder	2.8%
☐ oxides	3.0%
☐ acids	yes
☐ aromatic aldehydes	0.2%
☐ monoterpenes	24.0%
☐ alcohols	3.0%
☐ phenols,phe. ethers	62.0%

Stimulating   Balancing   Relaxing

BODY SYSTEMS

PROPERTIES > USES

NERVOUS SYSTEM
☐☐☐☐☐■

analgesic, antispasmodic, stimulant, tonic > gives strength and courage, paralysis, Raynaud's disease

ENDOCRINE SYSTEM
☐☐■■■

hormone like, oestrogen like, increases sweating >

CIRCULATION AND IMMUNE SYSTEM
☐☐☐■■■

bactericidal, decongestant, purifies, stimulant > angina, cardiac rhythm, palpitations

SKIN, MUSCLES AND BODY TISSUES
☐☐■■■■

antiinflammatory, antiseptic, insecticide > cellulite, dissolves boils and swellings, fluid retention, oedema, wrinkles

RESPIRATORY SYSTEM
☐☐☐■■■

decongestant, tonic > asthma, bronchitis, rapid breathing, whooping cough

DIGESTIVE SYSTEM
☐☐☐■■

bactericidal > anorexia, constipation, flatulence, indigestion, parasites

URINARY SYSTEM
☐☐■☐■■

diuretic > cystitis, infections, kidney stones

REPRODUCTIVE SYSTEM
☐☐☐■■

breast decongestant > amenorrhoea, assists childbirth, regulates menstrual cycle, stimulates milk production

CAUTIONS

Do not use with pregnant women, babies and young children. Do not use if epilepsy is suspected.

BOTANICAL FAMILY

Umbelliferae : this family generally aids digestion.

Herb: distilled crushed seeds : sweet aniseed like aroma : top - middle note.
Sweet fennel mimics oestrogen(8). Note bitter fennel comes from distilling the herb and crushed seeds and contains up to 22% ketones and is thus best avoided.
Chemical constituents may include:

☐ fenchone

☐ bergaptene, umbelliferone

☐ 1.8-cineole

☐ anisaldehyde

☐ anisic acid

☐ α-pinene, α-thujene, γ-terpinene, limonene, myrcene, phellandrene

■ fenchol

■ trans-anethole, methyl chavicol (estragole)

FIR NEEDLE SILVER
Abies alba

▪ esters	7.0%
▪ aliphatic aldehydes	yes
▪ sesquiterpenes	yes
▫ remainder	3.0%
▪ monoterpenes	90.0%

Stimulating   Balancing   Relaxing

BODY SYSTEMS

NERVOUS SYSTEM
■■

ENDOCRINE SYSTEM

CIRCULATION AND IMMUNE SYSTEM
■■

SKIN, MUSCLES and BODY TISSUES
■■■■

RESPIRATORY SYSTEM
■■■

DIGESTIVE SYSTEM

URINARY SYSTEM

REPRODUCTIVE SYSTEM

PROPERTIES > USES

analgesic, stimulant >

bactericidal, decongestant > arteries

antiseptic > arthritis, muscular aches and pains, rheumatism

bactericidal > bronchitis, catarrh

BOTANICAL FAMILY

Pinaceae : this family is highly antiseptic and generally aids respiratory problems.

Tree: distilled needles and twigs : fragrant and soothing aroma : middle note.
It is important to know the botanical specification as there are many firs whose constituents are different.

Chemical constituents may include:

■ bornyl acetate   ■ pinene, camphene, limonene

■ lauraldehyde, decylaldehyde

FRANKINCENSE
Boswellia carteri

■	esters	yes
☐	ketones	yes
■	sesquiterpenes	yes
☐	remainder	60.0%
■	monoterpenes	40.0%
■	alcohols	yes

Stimulating   Balancing   Relaxing

BODY SYSTEMS	PROPERTIES > USES
NERVOUS SYSTEM ■■■■■	analgesic, antispasmodic, calming > helpful for anxious obsessional links to the past, postnatal depression
ENDOCRINE SYSTEM ☐☐☐■	regulates secretions >
CIRCULATION AND IMMUNE SYSTEM ■■■■■	astringent, bactericidal > cancer, immune stimulant, slows breathing
SKIN, MUSCLES and BODY TISSUES ■■■■■	antiinflammatory, antioxidant, cell regenerator > carbuncles, combats aging skin, ulcers, wounds, wrinkles
RESPIRATORY SYSTEM ■■■■■	expectorant, mucolytic > asthma, bronchitis, catarrh
DIGESTIVE SYSTEM ■■■■■	calming > flatulence, nephritis
URINARY SYSTEM ■■■■■	bactericidal > cystitis
REPRODUCTIVE SYSTEM ■■■■■	antiinflammatory > breast inflammation, genital infections, leucorrhoea

BOTANICAL FAMILY   Buseraceae.

Tree: distilled gum resin : woody spicy aroma : base note.
Historically used as incense and aid to meditation. It was burnt to banish evil spirits from sickrooms. Considered as precious as gold in Christ's time. Chinese treated TB of lympth glands with it. Slows breathing pace(9). Extremely variable composition.

Chemical constituents may include:

■ octyl acetate

■ guaiene, copaene,
   trans-caryophyllene

■ α-pinene, β-pinene, α-terpinene, dipentene,
   p-cymene, thujene, myrcene, phellandrene,
   limonene

■ octanol, farnesol

GERANIUM
Pelargonium graveolens

■ esters	15.0%
■ aliphatic aldehydes	5.0%
□ ketones	7.0%
■ sesquiterpenes	4.0%
□ remainder	2.0%
□ oxides	2.0%
■ monoterpenes	2.0%
■ alcohols	63.0%

Stimulating   Balancing   Relaxing

BODY SYSTEMS

NERVOUS SYSTEM
■■■■■

ENDOCRINE SYSTEM
■■■■

CIRCULATION AND IMMUNE SYSTEM
■■■■□■■

SKIN, MUSCLES and BODY TISSUES
■■■■□■■

RESPIRATORY SYSTEM
■■■■■

DIGESTIVE SYSTEM
■■■■□■■

URINARY SYSTEM
■■■■□■■

REPRODUCTIVE SYSTEM
■■■■■

SUMMARY

BOTANICAL FAMILY

PROPERTIES > USES

analgesic, antispasmodic, calming > anxiety, nervous fatigue, neuralgia, Raynaud's disease

balancing, regulates hormone function > acts on the adrenal cortex

anticoagulant, bactericidal, tonic > constricts blood vessels, fluid retention, stems bleeding, varicose veins

antifungal, antiinflammatory, antioxidant, antiseptic, cell regenerator > athlete's foot, burns, haemorrhoids, impetigo, rheumatism

bactericidal > tonsillitis

decongestant, stimulant > diabetes, diarrhoea, colitis, gall bladder, jaundice, liver, pancreas

diuretic > cystitis, kidney stones

decongestant > breast congestion, candida, painful periods, pmt, uterine haemorrhage

Excellent all round balancer, eliminates waste and congestion.

Geraniaceae.

Plant 60cm perennial: distilled leaves and flowers : sweet rose like aroma : middle note. Traditionally a great healing plant often planted around dwellings to ward off evil spirits. Tests show strong bactericidal action(10).

Chemical constituents may include:

■ citronellyl formate, geranyl formate

■ citral

□ menthone

■ guaiazulene, β-caryophyllene

□ cis-rose oxide

■ phellandrene, limonene, α-pinene

■ citronellol, geraniol, linalool

GINGER
Zingiber officinale

	esters	2.0%
	aliphatic aldehydes	5.0%
	ketones	2.0%
	sesquiterpenes	55.0%
	remainder	4.7%
	oxides	1.3%
	monoterpenes	20.0%
	alcohols	10.0%

Stimulating   Balancing   Relaxing

BODY SYSTEMS	PROPERTIES > USES
NERVOUS SYSTEM	analgesic, antispasmodic, aphrodisiac, cheering > neuralgia
ENDOCRINE SYSTEM	causes sweating, temperature reducing >
CIRCULATION AND IMMUNE SYSTEM	stimulant > angina, cholesterol, varicose veins
SKIN, MUSCLES and BODY TISSUES	antioxidant, antiseptic > arthritis, back spasms, hearing, lower toothache, rheumatism, sight
RESPIRATORY SYSTEM	expectorant > catarrh, chronic bronchitis, good for all side effects of colds
DIGESTIVE SYSTEM	stimulant, tonic > constipation, diarrhoea, hangover, indigestion, flatulence, nausea, seasickness
URINARY SYSTEM	
REPRODUCTIVE SYSTEM	balancing > disperses clots, helpful after childbirth

BOTANICAL FAMILY	Zingiberaceae.

Herb: distilled unpeeled dried ground rhizome : warm pleasant spicy aroma : top note.
Used in many ancient remedies. Prevents stomach griping when added to purgatives(11).

Chemical constituents may include:

- geranial, citronellal
- gingerone
- β-sesquiphellandrene, zingiberene, *ar*-curcumene

- 1.8-cineole
- α-pinene, β-pinene, camphene, limonene, phellandrene
- citronellol, linalool, borneol, gingerol

34

GRAPEFRUIT
Citrus paradisi

■	esters	0.5%
■	aliphatic aldehydes	1.5%
□	ketones	yes
▨	sesquiterpenes	yes
▨	lactones and coumarins	0.5%
□	remainder	0.5%
▨	monoterpenes	96.0%
■	alcohols	1.0%

Stimulating   Balancing   Relaxing

BODY SYSTEMS	PROPERTIES > USES

NERVOUS SYSTEM
■ ■ □ ■ ■ ■

calming > relieves stress headaches and migraine

ENDOCRINE SYSTEM
□ ■

secretions > gall and liver

CIRCULATION AND IMMUNE SYSTEM
■ □ ■

antiviral > colds and flu

SKIN, MUSCLES and BODY TISSUES
■ ■ □ ■ ■ ■

air antiseptic > local infections, treats congested skin

RESPIRATORY SYSTEM

DIGESTIVE SYSTEM
□ ■

secretions > breaks up gall stones, liver problems

URINARY SYSTEM
□ ■ ■

diuretic >

REPRODUCTIVE SYSTEM

NOTE   Unlike other citrus oils grapefruit oil is not phototoxic.

BOTANICAL FAMILY   Rutaceae : this family generally aids digestion and skin.

Tree: expressed from peel of fruit : sharp refreshing aroma : top note.
Used widely in foods and cosmetics. It is liable to oxidise quickly.

Chemical constituents may include:

■ geranyl acetate   □ auraptene, limettin

■ citronellal, citral, sinensal   □ limonene

□ cadinene   ■ paradisiol, geraniol

35

HYSSOP
Hyssopus officinalis

■ esters	2.0%
□ ketones	46.0%
■ sesquiterpenes	8.0%
□ remainder	3.2%
□ oxides	0.8%
□ acids	yes
■ monoterpenes	28.0%
■ alcohols	8.0%
■ phenols,phe. ethers	4.0%

Stimulating   Balancing   Relaxing

BODY SYSTEMS

NERVOUS SYSTEM
■■■□□■■

ENDOCRINE SYSTEM
□■

CIRCULATION AND IMMUNE SYSTEM
■■□□■■

SKIN, MUSCLES and BODY TISSUES
■■□□□■■■

RESPIRATORY SYSTEM
■■■□□■■■

DIGESTIVE SYSTEM
■■■□■■■

URINARY SYSTEM
■■■□■■■

REPRODUCTIVE SYSTEM
□□■

CAUTIONS

BOTANICAL FAMILY

PROPERTIES > USES

antispasmodic, sedative > clears head, grief, multiple sclerosis, releases emotional pain

stimulates sweating > stimulates menstrual flow

astringent, bactericidal, decongestant, regulates blood pressure > cardiac

antiinflammatory, antiseptic > bruises, dissolves boils and swellings, rheumatism, rhinopharyngitis, sinusitis

expectorant > asthma, bronchitis, catarrh, colds, chest infections, coughs, emphysema, hayfever

tonic > digestion heavy fats, flatulence, indigestion, intestinal parasites

diuretic > cystitis, kidney stones

emmenagogue > leucorrhoea

Avoid in cases of pregnancy and epilepsy.

Lamiaceae.

Herb: distilled flowering tops and leaves : warm herby penetrating aroma : middle note. Historically renowned for its cleansing properties possible help for cancer.

Chemical constituents may include:

- ■ bornyl acetate, methyl myrtenate
- □ pinocamphone, isopinocamphone, camphor
- ■ caryophyllene, cadinene
- □ 1.8-cineole, caryophyllene oxide
- ■ β-pinene, camphene, limonene, myrcene, cis-ocimene
- ■ borneol, geraniol, linalool
- ■ methyl chavicol (estragole)

36

JASMIN
Jasminum officinale

■ esters	54.0%
■ ketones	2.7%
☐ remainder	16.6%
☐ acids	yes
■ aromatic aldehydes	yes
■ alcohols	24.0%
■ phenols,phe. ethers	2.7%

Stimulating   Balancing   Relaxing

BODY SYSTEMS

PROPERTIES > USES

NERVOUS SYSTEM
■ ■ ■ ■ ■

antispasmodic, aphrodisiac, calming, sedative > depression, restores confidence and thus energises

ENDOCRINE SYSTEM
■ ■ ■

hormone like > stimulates milk production, stimulates uterine muscles in childbirth, useful after childbirth

CIRCULATION AND IMMUNE SYSTEM

SKIN, MUSCLES and BODY TISSUES
■ ■ ☐ ■ ■ ■

antiseptic > good skin balm, relaxes muscles, stretch marks

RESPIRATORY SYSTEM
■ ■ ■ ■

antispasmodic > calms coughs, regulates and deepens breathing, relieves bronchial spasms

DIGESTIVE SYSTEM

URINARY SYSTEM

REPRODUCTIVE SYSTEM
■ ■ ■ ■

uterine tonic > hastens birth delivery, increases milk supply, increases sperm count, vaginal infections

CAUTIONS

Do not use during pregnancy.

BOTANICAL FAMILY

Oleaceae.

Shrub: solvent extraction from flowers : exotic flowery heady aroma : base note. Considered to be the ' king' of flower oils long used in love potions.

Chemical constituents may include:

■ benzyl acetate, linalyl acetate, benzyl benzoate, methyl jasmonate, methyl anthranilate

☐ cis-jasmone

☐ indole

☐ phenylacetic acid

■ linalool, nerol, geraniol, benzyl alcohol, farnesol, terpineol, phytols

■ eugenol

JUNIPER BERRY
Juniperus communis

■ esters	yes
■ sesquiterpenes	6.0%
■ lactones and coumarins	yes
□ remainder	9.0%
□ oxides	yes
■ acids	yes
■ monoterpenes	80.0%
■ alcohols	5.0%

Stimulating   Balancing   Relaxing

BODY SYSTEMS | **PROPERTIES > USES**

NERVOUS SYSTEM
■ ■ ■ ■
analgesic, antispasmodic, aphrodisiac > insomnia, sciatica

ENDOCRINE SYSTEM
□ □ ■
causes sweating, controls sebum production, regulates menstrual cycle, stimulates secretions >

CIRCULATION AND IMMUNE SYSTEM
□ □ ■
antiseptic >

SKIN, MUSCLES and BODY TISSUES
■ ■ ■ □ □ ■ ■
antiseptic > cellulite, fluid retention, eliminates uric acid, obesity, oedema, painful joints, psoriasis, stiffness

RESPIRATORY SYSTEM

DIGESTIVE SYSTEM
■ ■ ■ □ □ ■
stimulates secretions > cirrhosis, clears mucous from intestines, diabetes, liver, pancreas, stimulates appetite

URINARY SYSTEM
■ ■ □ ■ ■
diuretic > cystitis, kidney stones, prostate, strangury (unable to pass urine)

REPRODUCTIVE SYSTEM
□ □ ■
regulates > amenorrhoea, assists childbirth, menstrual

CAUTIONS
Avoid in pregnancy. Do not use if kidneys are inflammed.

BOTANICAL FAMILY
Cupressaceae : this family generally aids nervous tension, rheumatism and cellulite.

Shrub: distilled berries : fresh woody aroma : middle note.
Used medicinally for urinary infections. Expels uric acid from the system and is a powerful detoxifying agent.
Chemical constituents may include:

■ bornyl acetate, terpinyl acetate

□ caryophyllene oxide

■ caryophyllene, cadinene, humulene, germacrene

■ α-pinene, β-pinene, γ-terpinene, p-cymene, limonene, sabinene, thujene, myrcene, camphene

■ umbelliferone

■ terpinen-4-ol, α-terpineol

JUNIPER TWIGS
Juniperus communis

■	esters	yes
■	sesquiterpenes	3.0%
■	lactones and coumarins	yes
□	remainder	19.0%
□	acids	yes
■	monoterpenes	75.0%
■	alcohols	3.0%

Stimulating   Balancing   Relaxing

BODY SYSTEMS	PROPERTIES > USES
NERVOUS SYSTEM ■■■■	analgesic, antispasmodic, neurotonic > mental fatigue
ENDOCRINE SYSTEM ■	reduces production of sebum >
CIRCULATION AND IMMUNE SYSTEM ■□■	antiseptic, decongestant > arteriosclerosis
SKIN, MUSCLES and BODY TISSUES ■■■□■■	antiinflammatory > rheumatism, fluid retention, gout, greasy hair, weeping eczema
RESPIRATORY SYSTEM ■■■■	expectorant > bronchitis, catarrh, rhinitis
DIGESTIVE SYSTEM	
URINARY SYSTEM ■■□■■	diuretic > cystitis, kidney stones, prostate block, strangury (unable to pass urine)
REPRODUCTIVE SYSTEM	
CAUTIONS	Avoid in preganacy. Do not use if kidneys are inflamed.
BOTANICAL FAMILY	Cupressaceae : this family generally aids nervous tension, rheumatism and cellulite.

Shrub: distilled twigs : fresh terpentine like aroma : middle note.
Celtic junepurs means acrid or biting. Juniper twigs were burned to purify air in hospitals.
Famous as an ingredient of gin.
Chemical constituents may include:

■ β-caryophyllene   ■ terpinen-4-ol

□ α-pinene, β-pinene, γ-terpinene,
   limonene, myrcene, sabinene, thujene

LAVANDIN
Lavandula hybrida

■	esters	30.0%
■	aliphatic aldehydes	yes
◻	ketones	10.0%
■	sesquiterpenes	1.0%
▨	lactones and coumarins	yes
◻	remainder	3.0%
◻	oxides	5.0%
◻	acids	yes
▨	aromatic aldehydes	yes
▨	monoterpenes	6.0%
■	alcohols	45.0%
■	phenols,phe. ethers	yes

Stimulating   Balancing   Relaxing

BODY SYSTEMS

NERVOUS SYSTEM
■ ■ ■ ■ ▨ ■

ENDOCRINE SYSTEM

CIRCULATION AND IMMUNE SYSTEM
■ ■ ■ ◻ ■ ▨ ■ ■

SKIN, MUSCLES and BODY TISSUES
■ ■ ■ ■ ■ ▨ ■ ■

RESPIRATORY SYSTEM
■ ■ ■ ◻ ■ ▨ ■ ■

DIGESTIVE SYSTEM

URINARY SYSTEM

REPRODUCTIVE SYSTEM

PROPERTIES > USES

slightly antispasmodic, calming > anxiety, insomnia

bactericidal, lowers blood pressure, slightly decongestant, heart tonic > phlebitis

antifungal, antiinflammatory, antiseptic > allergies, cramps, dermatitis, relaxes muscles, wounds

bactericidal > colds, coughs, flu, sinusitis

BOTANICAL FAMILY   Lamiaceae.

Shrub: distilled flower stalks : strong lavender aroma : middle note.
Lavandin is good for circulation and respiratory and muscle problems.

Chemical constituents may include:

■ linalyl acetate, bornyl acetate
◻ camphor
■ caryophyllene

◻ 1,8-cineole
▨ camphene, limonene, ocimene
■ linalool, α-terpineol, geraniol, lavandulol

40

LAVENDER SPIKE
Lavandula lactifolia

■	esters	2.0%
■	ketones	15.0%
■	sesquiterpenes	3.0%
■	lactones and coumarins	0.2%
□	remainder	3.8%
□	oxides	34.0%
■	monoterpenes	10.0%
■	alcohols	32.0%

Stimulating   Balancing   Relaxing

BODY SYSTEMS

NERVOUS SYSTEM
■■■■□■■

ENDOCRINE SYSTEM
■■■

CIRCULATION AND IMMUNE SYSTEM
■■■■□■■

SKIN, MUSCLES and BODY TISSUES
■■■■□■■

RESPIRATORY SYSTEM
■■■■□■■

DIGESTIVE SYSTEM
■■■■■

URINARY SYSTEM

REPRODUCTIVE SYSTEM

PROPERTIES > USES

analgesic, antidepressant, calming > calms yet alerts, clears head, neuritis

regulating >

antiviral, bactericidal, decongestant, immune system tonic > cardiac

antifungal, antiseptic > acne, athlete's foot, bruises, midges, muscular aches and pains, rheumatism, ringworm

expectorant > bronchitis, catarrh, rhinitis

bactericidal > enteritis

BOTANICAL FAMILY   Lamiaceae.

Shrub: distilled flower stalks : fresh lavender with camphor tones aroma : middle note.
More aggressive oil than true lavender due to the high camphor and cineole constituents.

Chemical constituents may include:

- ■ linalyl acetate
- ■ camphor
- ■ caryophyllene

- □ 1.8-cineole
- ■ camphene, limonene
- ■ borneol, linalool, lavandulol

LAVENDER TRUE
Lavandula angustifolia

■ esters	45.0%
■ aliphatic aldehydes	1.0%
☐ ketones	4.0%
■ sesquiterpenes	5.0%
■ lactones and coumarins	0.3%
☐ remainder	1.7%
☐ oxides	2.0%
■ aromatic aldehydes	1.0%
■ monoterpenes	4.0%
■ alcohols	36.0%
■ phenols,phe. ethers	yes

Stimulating   Balancing   Relaxing

BODY SYSTEMS

NERVOUS SYSTEM
■■■■■☐■■■

ENDOCRINE SYSTEM
■■■■■■■■

CIRCULATION AND IMMUNE SYSTEM
■■■■■☐■■■

SKIN, MUSCLES AND BODY TISSUES
■■■■■■■

RESPIRATORY SYSTEM
■■■■■☐■■■

DIGESTIVE SYSTEM
■■■

URINARY SYSTEM
■■■■■■■

REPRODUCTIVE SYSTEM
■■■■■☐■■■

BOTANICAL FAMILY

PROPERTIES > USES

analgesic, antispasmodic, balancing, calming, cheering > anxiety, headaches, insomnia, migraines, Raynaud's disease

nervous system regulator (opposite in large doses) > stimulates menstrual cycle

antiviral, bactericidal, lowers blood pressure, mildly decongestant, heart tonic > phlebitis, varicose veins

antifungal, antiinflammatory, antiseptic, cell regenerator > arthritis, burns, radiography burns, eczema, herpes, psoriasis, spots, wounds

bactericidal > bronchitis, coughs, sinusitis, TB

stimulates, secretions > increases bile production, improves digestion heavy fats

bactericidal > cystitis

gentle emmenagogue > assists childbirth, candida, leucorrhoea, lower back massage helps expel afterbirth

Lamiaceae.

Shrub: distilled flower stalks : floral aroma : middle note.
Lavere means 'to wash'. Lavender was used extensively by the Romans in their baths.
Lavender oils exhibit antifungal properties(13),(14),(15).
Chemical constituents may include:

- ■ linalyl acetate, geranyl acetate, lavandulyl acetate
- ■ citral
- ☐ octanone, camphor
- ■ β-caryophyllene
- ■ terpinen-4-ol, α-terpineol, linalool, borneol, geraniol, lavandulol
- ■ coumarin, umbelliferone
- ☐ 1.8-cineole, linalool oxide, caryophyllene oxide
- ■ cuminaldehyde, benzaldehyde
- ■ ocimene, camphene, limonene

LEMON
Citrus limon

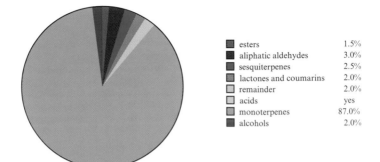

esters	1.5%
aliphatic aldehydes	3.0%
sesquiterpenes	2.5%
lactones and coumarins	2.0%
remainder	2.0%
acids	yes
monoterpenes	87.0%
alcohols	2.0%

  ●

Stimulating   Balancing   Relaxing

BODY SYSTEMS	PROPERTIES > USES
NERVOUS SYSTEM ■■■■	antispasmodic, calming and clarifying > headaches, insomnia, nightmares
ENDOCRINE SYSTEM	
CIRCULATION AND IMMUNE SYSTEM ■■■□■	antiviral, bactericidal, lowers blood pressure, decongestant, stimulant > cellulite, cleanses, obesity, stems bleeding
SKIN, MUSCLES and BODY TISSUES ■■■■□□■	antiaging, antifungal, antiseptic, skin tonic, phototoxic > arthritis, boils, brown patches, dry or aging skin, gout, rheumatism, verrucas, warts
RESPIRATORY SYSTEM ■■■□■	calming > bronchitis, catarrh
DIGESTIVE SYSTEM ■■■□	calming > diabetes, gall stones, liver, ulcers
URINARY SYSTEM □■	diuretic > kidney stones
REPRODUCTIVE SYSTEM ■■	antifungal > thrush
CAUTIONS	Phototoxic(1).
BOTANICAL FAMILY	Rutaceae : this family generally aids digestion and skin problems.

Tree: cold expression outer fresh peel : fresh sharp aroma : top note.
General rejuvenator due to its oxidising agents. Wide therapeutic values. D-limonene has been known to dissolve gall stones(11).
Chemical constituents may include:

- neryl acetate, geranyl acetate, terpinyl acetate
- citral, citronellal, nonanal, octanal, decanal
- β-bisabolene, α-bergamotene
- bergaptene, bergamottin

- limonene, α-pinene, β-pinene, γ-terpinene, camphene, phellandrene, p-cymene, sabinene, myrcene
- linalool, geraniol, octanol, α-terpineol, nonanol

43

LEMONGRASS EAST INDIAN
Cymbopogon flexuosus

■	esters	yes
■	aliphatic aldehydes	80.0%
■	ketones	yes
☐	remainder	3.0%
☐	acids	yes
■	monoterpenes	1.0%
■	alcohols	16.0%

Stimulating   Balancing   Relaxing

BODY SYSTEMS	PROPERTIES > USES
NERVOUS SYSTEM ■ ■ ☐ ■ ■	sedative, uplifting > depression
ENDOCRINE SYSTEM ☐ ☐ ■	milk flow, reduces sweating, stimulates secretions > stimulates para-sympathetic nerves
CIRCULATION AND IMMUNE SYSTEM ■ ☐ ☐ ■	bactericidal > arteries, stimulates circulation, vasodilatory
SKIN, MUSCLES and BODY TISSUES ■ ■ ☐ ☐ ■	antifungal, antiinflammatory, antiseptic, irritant, tissue toner > acne, athlete's foot, cellulite, eliminates lactic acid, fleas, pests, tired legs
RESPIRATORY SYSTEM	
DIGESTIVE SYSTEM ■ ■ ☐ ■	tonic > flatulence, liver
URINARY SYSTEM ☐ ☐ ■	diuretic >
REPRODUCTIVE SYSTEM ☐	stimulates secretions > stimulates milk flow
CAUTIONS	Possible skin irritation.
BOTANICAL FAMILY	Gramineae : this family generally aids aches and pains and stimulates circulation.

Grass: distilled fresh partially dried leaves : sweet strong lemon aroma : top note. Used in traditional Indian medicine for fevers and infections also considered to be a sedative to the central nervous system. Might arrest growth of tumours.

Chemical constituents may include:

■ citral

☐ methyl heptenone

☐ limonene, dipentene,

■ borneol, geraniol, nerol, farnesol, terpineol

LEMONGRASS WEST INDIAN
Cymbopogon citratus

■	esters	yes
■	aliphatic aldehydes	80.0%
□	ketones	0.3%
■	sesquiterpenes	1.0%
□	remainder	3.7%
□	acids	yes
■	monoterpenes	14.0%
■	alcohols	1.0%

Stimulating   Balancing   Relaxing

BODY SYSTEMS	PROPERTIES > USES
NERVOUS SYSTEM ■■□■■■	sedative, uplifting > depression
ENDOCRINE SYSTEM □□■	milk flow, reduces sweating, stimulates secretions > stimulates para-sympathetic nerves
CIRCULATION AND IMMUNE SYSTEM ■■■■	bactericidal > arteries, stimulates circulation, vasodilatory
SKIN, MUSCLES and BODY TISSUES ■■□■■	antifungal, antiinflammatory, antiseptic, calming, irritant, tissue toner > acne, athlete's foot, cellulite, eliminates lactic acid, fleas, pests, tired legs
RESPIRATORY SYSTEM	
DIGESTIVE SYSTEM ■■□■■	tonic > flatulence, liver
URINARY SYSTEM □□■	diuretic >
REPRODUCTIVE SYSTEM □	stimulates secretions > stimulates milk flow
CAUTIONS	Possible skin irritation.
BOTANICAL FAMILY	Gramineae : this family generally aids aches and pains and stimulates circulation.

Grass: distilled fresh partially dried leaves : sweet strong lemon aroma : top note.
Used traditionally for fevers and infections. Widely used in perfumes and flavourings.
Similar properties to east indian lemongrass: found effective against tinea(16). There are many chemotypes.

Chemical constituents may include:

■ citral

□ methyl heptenone

□ mycrene, dipentene

■ linalool, geraniol, nerol, citronellol, farnesol

LIME
Citrus aurantifolia

esters	7.0%
aliphatic aldehydes	13.0%
sesquiterpenes	yes
lactones and coumarins	2.0%
remainder	2.0%
oxides	yes
monoterpenes	72.0%
alcohols	4.0%

Stimulating   Balancing   Relaxing

BODY SYSTEMS	PROPERTIES > USES
NERVOUS SYSTEM ■■■■■	antispasmodic, sedative > anxiety, stress
ENDOCRINE SYSTEM ■■	temperature control > cooling
CIRCULATION AND IMMUNE SYSTEM ■■■□□■■	anticoagulant, antiviral, bactericidal, lowers blood pressure, tonic > stems bleeding
SKIN, MUSCLES and BODY TISSUES ■■■■□□□	antiinflammatory, antiseptic, phototoxic > possible irritant, rheumatism, scurvy
RESPIRATORY SYSTEM ■■■□□■	decongestant, mucolytic > catarrh, sinusitis
DIGESTIVE SYSTEM ■■□□■	stimulant > calms digestion, stimulates appetite
URINARY SYSTEM	
REPRODUCTIVE SYSTEM	
CAUTIONS	Phototoxic(1).
BOTANICAL FAMILY	Rutaceae : this family generally aids digestion and skin.

Tree: cold expression of peel of unripe fruit : fresh sweet aroma : top note.
Lime oil that is distilled from the crushed fruit contains lower percentages of esters and aldehydes and only traces, if that, of the coumarins. Distilled oil has a sharp fresh aroma.

Chemical constituents may include:

■ geranyl acetate, methyl anthranilate

■ citral

■ bisabolene

■ bergaptene, limettin

■ limonene, pinenes, camphene, terpinolene, sabinene, p-cymene, myrcene

■ α-terpineol, linalool

MANDARIN
Citrus reticulata

■ esters	1.0%
■ aliphatic aldehydes	1.0%
■ lactones and coumarins	yes
☐ remainder	3.0%
■ monoterpenes	90.0%
■ alcohols	5.0%
■ phenols,phe. ethers	yes

Stimulating   Balancing   Relaxing

BODY SYSTEMS	PROPERTIES > USES
NERVOUS SYSTEM ■ ■ ■	antispasmodic, revitalising > anxiety, insomnia
ENDOCRINE SYSTEM ■ ■ ■	stimulates secretions > balances metabolic rate, bile
CIRCULATION AND IMMUNE SYSTEM ■ ☐ ■ ■	antiviral, tonic >
SKIN, MUSCLES and BODY TISSUES ■ ☐ ■ ■	antiseptic, cell regenerator > excellent for stretch marks
RESPIRATORY SYSTEM	
DIGESTIVE SYSTEM ■ ■ ☐	calming > breaks down fats, flatulence, improves bile production, liver
URINARY SYSTEM	
REPRODUCTIVE SYSTEM	
NOTE	Especially good for children, women and elderly.
BOTANICAL FAMILY	Rutaceae : this family generally aids digestion and skin.

Tree: cold expression of the outer peel : sweet sharp floral aroma : top note.
This fruit was given to the Mandarins as a mark of respect - hence its name.

Chemical constituents may include:

- ■ methyl anthranilate
- ■ decanal, sinensal, citral, citronellal
- ☐ γ-terpinene, limonene, pinenes, myrcene, p-cymene
- ■ linalool, citronellol, octanol
- ■ thymol

MARJORAM SPANISH
Thymus mastichina

■ esters	5.0%
■ ketones	4.0%
■ sesquiterpenes	1.0%
☐ remainder	2.0%
☐ oxides	55.0%
■ monoterpenes	9.0%
■ alcohols	20.0%
■ phenols,phe. ethers	4.0%

Stimulating   Balancing   Relaxing

BODY SYSTEMS	PROPERTIES > USES
NERVOUS SYSTEM ■■■	calming >
ENDOCRINE SYSTEM ■■■	stimulates mucous glands, stimulates secretions >
CIRCULATION AND IMMUNE SYSTEM ■■■■	bactericidal >
SKIN, MUSCLES and BODY TISSUES ■■■■■	antiseptic >
RESPIRATORY SYSTEM ■■☐■■■	decongestant, expectorant > stimulates mucous glands
DIGESTIVE SYSTEM	
URINARY SYSTEM	
REPRODUCTIVE SYSTEM	

BOTANICAL FAMILY   Lamiaceae.

Herb: distilled dried flowering herb : musty herby aroma : middle note.
There is considerable confusion between species of oregano and majoram. Spanish majoram has a different botanical classification to the french majoram.

Chemical constituents may include:

■ linalyl acetate, terpinyl acetate, *trans*-pinocarvyl acetate
■ camphor
■ β-caryophyllene, gurjunene
☐ 1.8-cineole, caryophyllene oxide

☐ α-pinene, β-pinene, α-terpinene, γ-terpinene, limonene, *p*-cymene, terpinolene

■ linalool, α-terpineol, *cis*-thujanol, *trans*-thujanol, *trans*-pinocarveol

■ thymol

MARJORAM SWEET
Origanum majorana

esters	2.0%
aliphatic aldehydes	1.0%
sesquiterpenes	3.0%
remainder	4.0%
monoterpenes	40.0%
alcohols	50.0%
phenols,phe. ethers	yes

Stimulating   Balancing   Relaxing

BODY SYSTEMS

NERVOUS SYSTEM
■■■□■■

ENDOCRINE SYSTEM
■■□■■

CIRCULATION AND IMMUNE SYSTEM
■■□■■

SKIN, MUSCLES and BODY TISSUES
■■□■■■

RESPIRATORY SYSTEM
■■■□■■

DIGESTIVE SYSTEM
■■■□■■

URINARY SYSTEM

REPRODUCTIVE SYSTEM
■□■■

CAUTIONS

BOTANICAL FAMILY

PROPERTIES > USES

analgesic, aphrodisiac, antispasmodic, balancing, calming > addiction, depression, headaches, obsessional, psychoses, vertigo

balances > para-sympathetic nerves, under active thyroid

antiviral, bactericidal, lowers blood pressure > arteries, balances heart and circulation, vasodilatory

antifungal, antioxidant, antiseptic > arthritis, bruises (due to blood flow), cuts, muscle aches, rheumatism, toothache

bactericidal > bronchitis, catarrh, colds, coughs, nervous breathing, otitis, rhinitis, sinusitis

calming, diuretic > diarrhoea, enteritis, flatulence, laxative, ulcers

emmenagogue > painful periods, sexual obsession problems

Avoid during pregnancy.

Lamiaceae.

Herb: distilled flowering herb : spicy warm camphor like aroma : middle note.
Powerful effect for hyperactivity, calming to the nervous system excellent for deep emotional traumas - grief, loneliness etc. There are many species of marjoram with classification origanum - very difficult to identify and name. Known as ' joy of the mountain', given to married couples and planted in graveyards to bring peace to the departed.

Chemical constituents may include:

■ linalyl acetate, terpinyl acetate, geranyl acetate

■ citral

■ caryophyllene, cadinene

■ β-pinene, α-terpinene, γ-terpinene, p-cymene, myrcene, limonene, ocimene, sabinene

■ linalool, borneol, α-terpineol, terpinen-4-ol

■ carvacrol, eugenol

MELISSA LEMON BALM
Melissa officinalis

■ esters	1.2%	
■ aliphatic aldehydes	50.0%	
☐ ketones	7.0%	
■ sesquiterpenes	20.0%	
■ lactones and coumarins	yes	
☐ remainder	11.8%	
☐ oxides	4.0%	
■ monoterpenes	1.0%	
■ alcohols	5.0%	

Stimulating   Balancing   Relaxing

BODY SYSTEMS

PROPERTIES > USES

NERVOUS SYSTEM
■ ■ ■ ■ ■ ☐ ■ ■

antispasmodic, calming central system, hypnotic, sedative > depression, grief, headaches, hysteria, insomnia, vertigo

ENDOCRINE SYSTEM
■ ■ ■ ■ ■ ■ ■

lowers fever, increases sweating > regulates heart, menstrual cycle and bile production

CIRCULATION AND IMMUNE SYSTEM
■ ■ ■ ☐ ■

lowers blood pressure > anaemia, angina, irregular heart beat , palpitations

SKIN, MUSCLES and BODY TISSUES
■ ■ ■ ■ ■ ■

antiinflammatory, possible irritant > herpes (reduces healing time and lengthens time between attacks), wasp and bee stings

RESPIRATORY SYSTEM
■ ■ ■ ■ ■ ☐ ☐

calming > allergies, rapid breathing

DIGESTIVE SYSTEM
■ ■ ■ ■ ■ ☐ ☐

calming > cramps, indigestion, liver, nausea

URINARY SYSTEM

REPRODUCTIVE SYSTEM
☐ ■ ■

uterine tonic >

CAUTIONS

Best avoided in pregnancy. Possible skin irritation. This oil is often adulterated.

BOTANICAL FAMILY

Lamiaceae.

Herb: distilled leaves and flowering tops : sweet lemon flowery aroma : middle note. Famous for its calming effect on the heart and its rejuvenating effect. Found to be relaxant(17). Most melissa oils sold are blends of oils as true melissa is extremely expensive.

Chemical constituents may include:

■ geranyl acetate, neryl acetate, citronellyl acetate
■ citronellal, citral
☐ methyl heptenone
■ β-caryophyllene, germacrene, α-copaene

☐ 1.8-cineole, caryophyllene oxide
■ limonene, *trans*-ocimene
■ citronellol, geraniol, linalool

MINT BERGAMOT
Mentha citrata

■ esters	60.0%
■ aliphatic aldehydes	yes
■ sesquiterpenes	0.9%
☐ remainder	6.2%
☐ oxides	3.0%
☐ acids	yes
■ monoterpenes	0.9%
■ alcohols	29.0%

Stimulating   Balancing   Relaxing

BODY SYSTEMS	PROPERTIES > USES
NERVOUS SYSTEM ■ ■ ■ ☐ ■ ■	antispasmodic, tonic > nervous exhaustion, soothing
ENDOCRINE SYSTEM ■ ■ ■ ☐	balancing > stimulates liver and pancreas secretions
CIRCULATION AND IMMUNE SYSTEM ■ ■ ☐ ■ ■	slightly bactericidal > heart regulation
SKIN, MUSCLES and BODY TISSUES ■ ■ ■ ■ ■	slightly antiseptic, parasiticide > soothing
RESPIRATORY SYSTEM	
DIGESTIVE SYSTEM ☐ ■	parasiticide, stimulates secretions > gastric, liver, pancreas
URINARY SYSTEM ■ ■ ■ ■ ■	bactericidal > cystitis
REPRODUCTIVE SYSTEM ■ ■ ■ ☐ ■	tonic > impotence, stimulates ovaries

BOTANICAL FAMILY   Lamiaceae.

Herb: distilled leaves and flowering tops : lemony mint aroma : middle note.
This mint has a high proportion of esters making it a gentler oil, excellent for balancing the body.

Chemical constituents may include:

■ linalyl acetate, geranyl acetate	☐ β-pinene
■ caryophyllene, germacrene	■ linalool, α-terpineol, citronellol, geraniol
☐ 1.8-cineole, *cis*-linalool oxide, *trans*-linalool oxide	

MINT CORNMINT
Mentha arvensis

esters	1.0%
aliphatic aldehydes	yes
ketones	20.0%
sesquiterpenes	1.0%
lactones and coumarins	yes
remainder	1.0%
oxides	yes
acids	yes
monoterpenes	6.0%
alcohols	70.0%
phenols,phe. ethers	1.0%

Stimulating   Balancing   Relaxing

BODY SYSTEMS	PROPERTIES > USES
NERVOUS SYSTEM	anaesthetic, antispasmodic, stimulant, tonic > agitation, depression, migraine, motor nerves, sciatica, trembling
ENDOCRINE SYSTEM	stimulates secretions > digestive juices, bile, gastric
CIRCULATION AND IMMUNE SYSTEM	bactericidal > energises heart
SKIN, MUSCLES and BODY TISSUES	antiseptic, antimicrobic > eczema, possible irritation, toothache
RESPIRATORY SYSTEM	expectorant > laryngitis, rhinitis, sinusitis
DIGESTIVE SYSTEM	bactericidal > flatulence, indigestion, liver, ulcers, vomiting, worms
URINARY SYSTEM	tonic > kidney, nephritis
REPRODUCTIVE SYSTEM	
CAUTIONS	Not for children under three years. Check for dermal irritation.
BOTANICAL FAMILY	Lamiaceae.

Herb: distilled flowering herb : sweet bitter minty aroma : top note.
Many practitioners prefer peppermint oil because commercial cornmint oil is often fractionated. Chinese medicine uses cornmint for earache, tumours and skin conditions.

Chemical constituents may include:

- menthyl acetate
- menthone, isomenthone, piperitone, thujone
- caryophyllene
- menthofuran
- limonene, pinene, phellandrene
- menthol

MINT PEPPERMINT
Mentha piperita

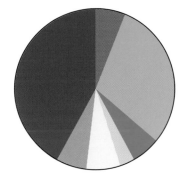

■ esters	6.0%
■ aliphatic aldehydes	yes
□ ketones	30.0%
■ sesquiterpenes	6.0%
■ lactones and coumarins	yes
□ remainder	3.0%
□ oxides	7.0%
□ acids	yes
■ monoterpenes	6.0%
■ alcohols	42.0%

Stimulating   Balancing   Relaxing

BODY SYSTEMS

NERVOUS SYSTEM
■ ■ ■ ■ ■ □ ■ ■

ENDOCRINE SYSTEM
■ ■ ■ ■ ■ □ ■ ■

CIRCULATION AND IMMUNE SYSTEM
□ ■ ■ ■

SKIN, MUSCLES and BODY TISSUES
■ ■ ■ ■ ■ □ ■

RESPIRATORY SYSTEM
■ ■ ■ ■ ■ □ ■

DIGESTIVE SYSTEM
■ ■ ■ ■ ■ □ ■

URINARY SYSTEM
■ ■ ■ ■ □ ■ ■ ■

REPRODUCTIVE SYSTEM
□ ■ □ □ ■

CAUTIONS

BOTANICAL FAMILY

PROPERTIES > USES

anaesthetic(18), analgesic, antispasmodic, tonic > mental fatigue, migraine, nervous trembling, sciatica

balancing, lowers fever, reduces milk production, lowers temperature > nervous system and menstrual cycle, stimulates heart and ovaries

antiviral, bactericidal, raises blood pressure > constricts capillaries

antifungal, antiinflammatory, antiseptic > asthma, eczema, gnats, herpes, rashes, ringworm, yellow fever

expectorant, mucolytic > bronchitis, laryngitis, otitis, rhinitis, sinusitis

tonic > cirrhosis, enteritis, gall stones, hepatitis, jaundice, liver, travel sickness, ulcers, vomiting, worms

bactericidal > cystitis, nephritis, prostate

uterine tonic > assists childbirth, impotence, reduces milk production

Not for use in pregnancy or with nursing mothers or with children under three years old.

Lamiaceae.

Herb: distilled leaves and flowering tops : piercing menthol aroma : top note.
Excellent for digestive problems and for local anaesthetic for wounds. Romans were well aware of its detoxifying properties and wore crowns of the herb at feasts. Used for irritable bowel syndrome(19).
Chemical constituents may include:

■ menthyl acetate

■ menthone, isomenthone, pulegone

■ germacrene, β-caryophyllene

■ aesculetine, menthofuran

□ 1.8-cineole, caryophyllene oxide

■ phellandrene, α-pinene, β-pinene, menthene, limonene

■ menthol, neomenthol, isomenthol, linalool

53

MINT SPEARMINT
Mentha spicata

■ esters	3.5%
■ ketones	55.0%
■ sesquiterpenes	3.0%
□ remainder	2.3%
□ oxides	2.2%
□ acids	yes
■ monoterpenes	12.0%
■ alcohols	22.0%

Stimulating   Balancing   Relaxing

BODY SYSTEMS	PROPERTIES > USES
NERVOUS SYSTEM ■■■□□■	calming, local anaesthetic, tonic > headaches, fatigue, migraine, nervous exhaustion, stress
ENDOCRINE SYSTEM □□■	lowers fever, lowers temperature, stimulates secretions > bile
CIRCULATION AND IMMUNE SYSTEM ■■□■■	decongestant, astringent >
SKIN, MUSCLES and BODY TISSUES ■■■□■■	antiseptic, strongly antiinflammatory > congested skin, wounds
RESPIRATORY SYSTEM ■■■□■	expectorant, mucolytic > bronchitis, fevers, flu, sinusitis
DIGESTIVE SYSTEM ■■■□■	tonic > bile flow, dyspepsia, flatulence, liver, vomiting
URINARY SYSTEM ■■■□□■	diuretic > cystitis

REPRODUCTIVE SYSTEM

CAUTIONS	Avoid in pregnancy and with young children.
BOTANICAL FAMILY	Lamiaceae.

Herb: distilled flowering tops : spicy warm minty aroma : top note.
Valued highly as a culinary herb. The water from distillation is used to relieve coughs, colic, hiccoughs and flatulence.

Chemical constituents may include:

■ *cis*-carvyl acetate, *trans*-carvyl acetate, dihydrocarvyl acetate

□ 1.8-cineole

■ carvone, dihydrocarvone, menthone

■ limonene, α-pinene, β-pinene phellandrene, camphene

■ caryophyllene, elemene, farnesene, bourbonene

■ linalool, menthol

MYRRH
Commiphora molmol

■	esters	yes
■	aliphatic aldehydes	2.0%
□	ketones	6.0%
■	sesquiterpenes	39.0%
□	remainder	10.0%
□	acids	yes
■	aromatic aldehydes	yes
□	monoterpenes	yes
■	alcohols	40.0%
■	phenols,phe. ethers	3.0%

Stimulating   Balancing   Relaxing

BODY SYSTEMS	PROPERTIES > USES
NERVOUS SYSTEM ■■□□□□■	calming > deodorant, sexual stimulus, weakness
ENDOCRINE SYSTEM ■□□■■	hormone like, temperature control > glandular fever, overactive thyroid
CIRCULATION AND IMMUNE SYSTEM ■■□■□	antiviral, astringent, bactericidal, immune system tonic > stimulates white corpuscles
SKIN, MUSCLES and BODY TISSUES ■■□□□□■	antifungal, antiinflammatory, antiseptic > athlete's foot, bedsores, gangrene, herpes, ringworm, ulcers, wet eczema
RESPIRATORY SYSTEM ■■□□□■■	antiseptic > bronchitis, drying nature excellent for pulmonary infections
DIGESTIVE SYSTEM ■■□□□■■	tonic > diarrhoea, haemorrhoids, hepatitis
URINARY SYSTEM □■■	diuretic >
REPRODUCTIVE SYSTEM ■■□□■■	emmenagogue > amenorrhoea, leucorrhoea, thrush

CAUTIONS   Best avoided in pregnancy.

BOTANICAL FAMILY   Buseraceae.

Tree: solvent extraction of crude myrrh to give a resinoid or steam distillation of the crude myrrh to give an essential oil : musky smoky aroma : base note.
Excellent for all septic skin conditions. Used in embalming.

Chemical constituents may include:

■ myrrholic ester,	□ myrrholic acid
■ 2-butanal	■ cinnamaldehyde, cuminaldehyde
□ methyl isobutyl ketone, curzerenone	■ limonene, dipentene, pinene
■ elemene, heerabolene, cadinene, copaene, curzerene, lindestrene	■ myrrh alcohols
	■ eugenol

NIAOULI
Melaleuca viridiflora

■ esters	15.0%
■ aliphatic aldehydes	yes
■ sesquiterpenes	yes
□ remainder	8.0%
□ oxides	60.0%
■ aromatic aldehydes	yes
■ monoterpenes	2.0%
■ alcohols	15.0%

Stimulating   Balancing   Relaxing

BODY SYSTEMS

PROPERTIES > USES

NERVOUS SYSTEM
■■■□■■■

analgesic, stimulant > aids concentration, clarifying

ENDOCRINE SYSTEM
■■■

lowers fever, oestrogen like >

CIRCULATION AND IMMUNE SYSTEM
■■□■■■

strongly antiviral, bactericidal, decongestant, immune system tonic > increases antibodies, HIV

SKIN, MUSCLES and BODY TISSUES
■■■□■■■

antiseptic, tissue toner > acne, aches and pains, boils, burns, radiography burns, rheumatism, spots, ulcers

RESPIRATORY SYSTEM
■■■□■■■

bactericidal > asthma, bronchitis, catarrh, coughs, pneumonia, sinusitis, sore throat

DIGESTIVE SYSTEM
■■□■■■

tonic > enteritis, gastric and duodenal ulcers, intestinal parasites

URINARY SYSTEM
■■■□■■■

bactericidal > cystitis

REPRODUCTIVE SYSTEM
■□■■■

antiviral > fibroids, genital herpes, leucorrhea, prostate

BOTANICAL FAMILY

Myrtaceae : this family is generally stimulating and good for the respiratory system.

Tree: distilled leaves and shoots : sweet clear penetrating aroma : top note.
Falling leaves cause healthy atmosphere due to strong disinfectant properties.
Recommended for serious conditions such as aids and nonhormonal cancer.

Chemical constituents may include:

■ terpinyl valerate, terpinyl acetate, terpinyl butyrate
■ isovaleraldehyde
■ β-caryophyllene, viridiflorene
□ 1.8-cineole

■ benzaldehyde

□ limonene, α-pinene, β-pinene

■ α-terpineol, viridiflorol, nerolidol, globulol

NUTMEG
Myristica fragrans

sesquiterpenes	1.0%
remainder	10.0%
oxides	2.0%
acids	yes
monoterpenes	75.0%
alcohols	6.0%
phenols,phe. ethers	6.0%

Stimulating   Balancing   Relaxing

BODY SYSTEMS

NERVOUS SYSTEM
■□□■■

ENDOCRINE SYSTEM
■■

CIRCULATION AND IMMUNE SYSTEM
■□■■■

SKIN, MUSCLES and BODY TISSUES
■□□■■■

RESPIRATORY SYSTEM

DIGESTIVE SYSTEM
□■■■

URINARY SYSTEM

REPRODUCTIVE SYSTEM
■□□■■

CAUTIONS

BOTANICAL FAMILY

PROPERTIES > USES

antispasmodic, tonic > excites motor cortex, neuralgia, Raynaud's disease

oestrogen like >

bactericidal > invigorating to heart and circulation

antiseptic, parasiticide > good for hair, haemorrhoids, rheumatism, sprains, toothache

stimulant > diarrhoea, digestion of heavy foods, gall stones

emmenagogue, uterine tonic > assists childbirth, frigidity, impotence, scanty periods

Treat with care the myristicin can cause hallucinations (20). Avoid in pregnancy.

Myristicaceae.

Tree: distilled fruits : sharp aroma : top note.
A nutmeg is like a small peach, the oil comes from the kernel. Oil obtained from the husk is called mace and contains even more myristicin. Nutmeg was traditionally used for stomach disorders. Nutmeg inhibits platelet aggregation(21).

Chemical constituents may include:

■ β-caryophyllene

□ 1.8-cineole

■ α-pinene, β-pinene, α-terpinene, γ-terpinene, sabinene, myrcene, limonene, camphene, dipentene, p-cymene

■ terpinen-4-ol, α-terpineol, linalool, borneol, geraniol

■ myristicin, elemicin, safrole, eugenol

ORANGE BITTER
Citrus aurantium amara

■	esters	2.0%
■	aliphatic aldehydes	2.0%
▩	ketones	yes
■	sesquiterpenes	0.5%
■	lactones and coumarins	0.5%
□	remainder	2.0%
□	oxides	yes
▢	acids	yes
▩	monoterpenes	90.0%
■	alcohols	3.0%

Stimulating   Balancing   Relaxing

BODY SYSTEMS

NERVOUS SYSTEM
■ ■ ■ ■ □ ■ ■

ENDOCRINE SYSTEM

CIRCULATION AND IMMUNE SYSTEM
■ ■ ■ □ ■ ■

SKIN, MUSCLES and BODY TISSUES
■ ■ ■ ■ ■ □ ■ ■

RESPIRATORY SYSTEM

DIGESTIVE SYSTEM
■ ■ ■ ■ ■ ■ ■

URINARY SYSTEM

REPRODUCTIVE SYSTEM

CAUTIONS

BOTANICAL FAMILY

PROPERTIES > USES

calming, cheering, stimulating > anxiety, vertigo

anticoagulant, bactericidal, astringent > circulation

antiaging, antifungal, antiinflammatory, antiseptic, cell regenerator, phototoxic, tonic >

calming > nervous indigestion, liver stimulant, constipation

Use with care skin may photosensitive after application(1).

Rutaceae : this family generally aids digestion and skin problems.

Tree: cold expression almost ripe peel : strong pervasive orange aroma : top note.
Both oranges and lemons have been used traditionally to treat palpitations, to thin the blood and to cure scurvy.
Chemical constituents may include:

■ linalyl acetate, geranyl acetate, citronellyl acetate

■ undecanal, citral

■ farnesene, copaene, humulene

■ auraptene, bergaptene, limettin

□ 1.8-cineole

▩ limonene, α-pinene, myrcene, terpinolene, camphene, p-cymene, ocimene

■ linalool, nerol, α-terpineol, citronellol

ORANGE BLOSSOM NEROLI
Citrus aurantium amara

■ esters	14.0%
■ aliphatic aldehydes	2.0%
□ ketones	0.5%
■ sesquiterpenes	yes
□ remainder	8.5%
□ acids	yes
■ monoterpenes	35.0%
■ alcohols	40.0%

Stimulating   Balancing   Relaxing

BODY SYSTEMS

PROPERTIES > USES

NERVOUS SYSTEM
■■□□■□■

analgesic, aphrodisiac, antispasmodic > peace inducing, revitalising

ENDOCRINE SYSTEM
■■□■■

balancing > menopause, pmt

CIRCULATION AND IMMUNE SYSTEM
■■□■□□

bactericidal, lowers blood pressure, tonic > phlebitis, ulcers, varicose veins

SKIN, MUSCLES and BODY TISSUES
■■□■□■■

antiaging, antifungal, cell generator > deodorant, protection from radiography burns, rheumatism

RESPIRATORY SYSTEM
□□■

bactericidal > bronchitis, TB

DIGESTIVE SYSTEM
■■□□■□■

calming, tonic > diabetes, haemorrhoids, liver, pancreas

URINARY SYSTEM

REPRODUCTIVE SYSTEM
■■□□■■

uterine tonic > menopause, pmt

BOTANICAL FAMILY

Rutaceae : this family generally aids digestion and skin problems.

Tree: distilled freshly picked flowers : haunting and beautiful aroma : base note.
Very powerful for emotional problems. Used by Italian Countess of Neroli, Anne Marie, to perfume her gloves and bathing water - hence the name. Good antifungal activities.

Chemical constituents may include:

■ methyl anthranilate, <u>linalyl acetate,</u> geranyl acetate, neryl acetate

□ jasmone

□ indole

□ phenylacetic acid

■ <u>limonene, β-pinene</u>

■ <u>linalool,</u> α-terpineol, <u>geraniol, nerol,</u> nerolidol, farnesol, benzyl alcohol, phenylether alcohol

ORANGE PETITGRAIN
Citrus aurantium amara

esters	55.0%
aliphatic aldehydes	yes
lactones and coumarins	0.5%
remainder	4.5%
acids	yes
monoterpenes	10.0%
alcohols	30.0%
phenols,phe. ethers	yes

Stimulating   Balancing   Relaxing

BODY SYSTEMS

NERVOUS SYSTEM
■■■■■

ENDOCRINE SYSTEM

CIRCULATION AND IMMUNE SYSTEM
□■■

SKIN, MUSCLES and BODY TISSUES
■■■□■■■

RESPIRATORY SYSTEM
■■■□■■■

DIGESTIVE SYSTEM
■■■■■

URINARY SYSTEM

REPRODUCTIVE SYSTEM

PROPERTIES > USES

antispasmodic, calming, cheering > depression, nervous exhaustion

bactericidal > slight stimulation of immune system

antifungal, antioxidant, antiseptic, deodorant > infected acne, rheumatism (nervous)

tonic > bronchitis

calming > flatulence, nervous indigestion

BOTANICAL FAMILY

Rutaceae : this family generally aids digestion and skin problems.

Tree: distilled leaves and twigs : woody floral aroma : top note.
Classic ingredient of eau-de-cologne and widely used as a food flavouring. Good antifungal agent(23).

Chemical constituents may include:

- ■ linalyl acetate, geranyl acetate , neryl acetate
- ■ citral
- □ limettin, bergaptene

- □ α–pinene, limonene, p-cymene, ocimene, myrcene
- ■ linalool, geraniol, nerolidol, α-terpineol
- ■ thymol

ORANGE SWEET
Citrus sinensis

aliphatic aldehydes	2.0%
ketones	2.0%
sesquiterpenes	yes
lactones and coumarins	0.5%
remainder	5.5%
acids	yes
monoterpenes	85.0%
alcohols	5.0%

Stimulating   Balancing   Relaxing

BODY SYSTEMS

PROPERTIES > USES

NERVOUS SYSTEM
■ ■ ■ ■ ■

sedative, warming > depression, nervous tension

ENDOCRINE SYSTEM
■ ■

stimulates secretions > bile

CIRCULATION AND IMMUNE SYSTEM
■ ■ ■ ■ ■

bactericidal, lowers blood pressure, stimulant > colds, flu, fluid retention, obesity

SKIN, MUSCLES and BODY TISSUES
■ ■ ■ ■ ■ ■

antifungal (22), antiinflammatory, antiseptic > dull complexion, mouth ulcers

RESPIRATORY SYSTEM
■ ■ ■ ■ ■

bactericidal, decongestant > bronchitis, chills

DIGESTIVE SYSTEM
■ ■ ■ ■ ■

carminative, tonic > bile flow, constipation, indigestion

URINARY SYSTEM

REPRODUCTIVE SYSTEM

BOTANICAL FAMILY

Rutaceae : this family generally aids digestion and skin problems.

Tree: cold expression of fresh peel or distilled fresh peel : lingering rich fruity aroma if expressed, a lighter aroma if distilled : top note.
Dried sweet orange peel is used in Chinese medicine.

Chemical constituents may include:

■ decanal, citronellal, octanal

□ carvone, α-ionone

■ bergaptene, auraptene

□ limonene, myrcene, sabinene, α-pinene

■ linalool, α-terpineol, geraniol

ORIGANUM
Origanum heracleoticum carvacroliferum

■	esters	3.5%
■	sesquiterpenes	yes
□	remainder	9.0%
□	oxides	0.3%
□	acids	yes
■	monoterpenes	12.0%
■	alcohols	0.2%
■	phenols,phe. ethers	75.0%

Stimulating   Balancing   Relaxing

BODY SYSTEMS	PROPERTIES > USES
NERVOUS SYSTEM ■■□■■■	analgesic, antispasmodic, stimulant, tonic > neuralgia
ENDOCRINE SYSTEM ■■	increases sweating > warming
CIRCULATION AND IMMUNE SYSTEM ■□■■■	antiviral, bactericidal > increases leucocyte activity, tonic to immune system
SKIN, MUSCLES and BODY TISSUES ■■□■■■■	antifungal, antiseptic, parasiticide > rheumatism, skin irritation possible
RESPIRATORY SYSTEM ■□■■■	expectorant > bronchitis, irritation of mucous membrane possible
DIGESTIVE SYSTEM ■■■	carminative > aerophagy (swallowing gulps of air), flatulence, worms
URINARY SYSTEM □■■	diuretic >
REPRODUCTIVE SYSTEM ■	emmenagogue >
CAUTIONS	Avoid in preganacy. Use with extreme care due to high percentage of phenols.
BOTANICAL FAMILY	Lamiaceae.

Herb: distilled dried flowering tops : herbaceous tarry refreshing aroma : middle note. Properties similar to common thyme (thymus vulgaris) and wild origanum (origanum vulgare) but has much higher percentage of phenols.

Chemical constituents may include:

■	linalyl acetate	□	α-terpinene, γ-terpinene, p-cymene
■	caryophyllene	■	linalool
□	1.8-cineole	■	carvacrol, thymol

PALMAROSA
Cymbopogon martinii

■	esters	5.0%
■	aliphatic aldehydes	7.0%
□	ketones	yes
■	sesquiterpenes	yes
□	remainder	3.0%
■	monoterpenes	yes
■	alcohols	85.0%

Stimulating   Balancing   Relaxing

BODY SYSTEMS

PROPERTIES > USES

NERVOUS SYSTEM
■ ■ ■ □ ■ ■

calming, cheering, tonic > nervous exhaustion

ENDOCRINE SYSTEM
■ □ ■ ■

lowers fever, stimulates sebum production > balances fluid retention

CIRCULATION AND IMMUNE SYSTEM
■ ■ □ ■ ■

strongly antiviral, antimicrobic, strongly bactericidal, tonic > cardiac

SKIN, MUSCLES and BODY TISSUES
■ ■ ■ ■ □ ■

strongly antifungal, antiseptic, cell generator > acne, dry cracked skin, dry and wet eczema, eases stiff joints

RESPIRATORY SYSTEM
■ ■ □ ■ ■

bactericidal > bronchitis, rhinitis, sinusitis

DIGESTIVE SYSTEM
■ ■ □ □ ■

stimulant > anorexia, enteritis

URINARY SYSTEM
■ ■ □ ■ ■ ■

bactericidal > cystitis

bactericidal > cystitis

REPRODUCTIVE SYSTEM
□ ■

uterine tonic > assists childbirth, cervix, uterus, vagina

BOTANICAL FAMILY

Gramineae : this family generally aids aches and pains and stimulates circulation.

Grass: distilled leaves : sweet dry rose like aroma : top note.
Known as Indian geranium oil, ginger grass is a chemotype of palmarosa. Often used to adulterate rose oil.

Chemical constituents may include:

- ■ geranyl acetate, geranyl formate, geranyl isobutyrate, geranyl hexanoate, neryl formate
- ■ citral, citronellal
- □ methyl heptenone

- ■ β-caryophyllene
- □ dipentene, limonene
- ■ geraniol, citronellol, farnesol, linalool, nerol, elemol

PATCHOULI
Pogostemon cablin

☐	ketones	2.0%
■	sesquiterpenes	50.0%
☐	remainder	8.0%
☐	oxides	6.0%
☐	acids	yes
■	monoterpenes	1.0%
■	alcohols	33.0%

Stimulating   Balancing   Relaxing

BODY SYSTEMS

PROPERTIES > USES

NERVOUS SYSTEM
■■□■■

aphrodisiac, balancing, calming, tonic > depression, makes mind more objective

ENDOCRINE SYSTEM
□■

lowers fever >

CIRCULATION AND IMMUNE SYSTEM
■■□■■

antiviral, astringent, bactericidal, decongestant, tonic to immune system > phlebitis, varicose veins

SKIN, MUSCLES and BODY TISSUES
■■□■■■

antifungal, antiinflammatory, antiseptic, cell generator > acne, athlete's foot, eczema, insects, loose or dry skin

RESPIRATORY SYSTEM

DIGESTIVE SYSTEM
■■□■■

carminative > curbs appetite, diarrhoea, enteritis, haemorrhoids

URINARY SYSTEM
□□■■

diuretic >

REPRODUCTIVE SYSTEM

BOTANICAL FAMILY   Lamiaceae.

Herb: distilled fermented dried leaves : sweet earthy aroma : base note.
Oil matures with age. Excellent for dry cracked skin conditions.

Chemical constituents may include:

☐ patchoulenone, isopatchoulenone

■ α-guaiene, patchoulenes, α-bulnesene, seychellenes, cadinene, caryophyllene, aromadendrene

☐ guaiene oxide, bulnesene oxide caryophyllene oxide

■ α-pinene, β-pinene, limonene

■ guaiol, bulnesol, pogostol, patchouli alcohol

PENNYROYAL
Mentha pulegium

esters	1.0%
ketones	80.0%
remainder	5.5%
monoterpenes	1.5%
alcohols	12.0%

Stimulating   Balancing   Relaxing

BODY SYSTEMS	PROPERTIES > USES
NERVOUS SYSTEM	antispasmodic, neurotoxic >
ENDOCRINE SYSTEM	lowers fever, causes sweating >
CIRCULATION AND IMMUNE SYSTEM	raises blood pressure > heart stimulant
SKIN, MUSCLES and BODY TISSUES	antiseptic > insect repellent
RESPIRATORY SYSTEM	mucolytic > bronchitis, catarrh
DIGESTIVE SYSTEM	carminative > flatulence, liver, spleen
URINARY SYSTEM	
REPRODUCTIVE SYSTEM	abortive, emmenagogue > leucorrhoea

CAUTIONS	Avoid in pregnancy and young children. Use with great caution as ketones can accumulate in the body.
BOTANICAL FAMILY	Lamiaceae.

Herb: distilled fresh or slightly dried herb : minty herby aroma.
Still in the British Herbal Pharmacopoeia for flatulence, intestinal colic, cutaneous eruptions, gout and delayed periods. Not recommended by some practitioners(24).

Chemical constituents may include:

- neoisomenthyl acetate
- pulegone, menthone, piperitenone, *trans*-isopulegone
- α-pinene, β-pinene, limonene
- linalool, menthol, neomenthol, neoisomenthol

PINE DWARF
Pinus mugo turra

■	esters	10.0%
■	aliphatic aldehydes	1.0%
■	ketones	1.0%
■	sesquiterpenes	1.0%
□	remainder	24.0%
■	aromatic aldehydes	1.0%
□	monoterpenes	60.0%
■	alcohols	2.0%

Stimulating   Balancing   Relaxing

BODY SYSTEMS	PROPERTIES > USES
NERVOUS SYSTEM ■■■■■	calming, cheering >
ENDOCRINE SYSTEM ■	slightly hormone like > warming
CIRCULATION AND IMMUNE SYSTEM ■■■■■	slightly bactericidal, slightly antiviral, decongestant > arteries, circulation
SKIN, MUSCLES and BODY TISSUES ■■■■■	slightly antiinflammatory, air antiseptic, irritant >
RESPIRATORY SYSTEM ■■■■■	antiseptic, expectorant > bronchitis, pleurisy, sinusitis, TB
DIGESTIVE SYSTEM	
URINARY SYSTEM ■■■	diuretic >
REPRODUCTIVE SYSTEM	
CAUTIONS	Use with care as skin irritation is likely. Some practitioners do not recommend the use of this oil.
BOTANICAL FAMILY	Pinaceae : this family is generally highly antiseptic and aids respiratory problems.

Tree: distilled needles and twigs : sweet soothing spicy woody unusual aroma due to aldehydes : middle note. The needles are used to make medical preparations for bladder, kidney and muscular pains also inhalents for respiratory problems.

Chemical constituents may include:

■ bornyl acetate, bornyl propionate, bornyl caproate
■ caproaldehyde
□ cryptone
■ cadinene

■ anisaldehyde, cuminaldehyde

□ Δ^3-carene, limonene, α-pinene, β-pinene phellandrene, myrcene, camphene, dipentene

■ pumiliol

PINE LONGLEAF TURPENTINE
Pinus palustris

esters	0.2%
remainder	2.6%
monoterpenes	96.0%
alcohols	1.0%
phenols,phe. ethers	0.2%

Stimulating   Balancing   Relaxing

BODY SYSTEMS

PROPERTIES > USES

NERVOUS SYSTEM
■ □ ■ ■

analgesic, antispasmodic, stimulant, warming > sciatica

ENDOCRINE SYSTEM

CIRCULATION AND IMMUNE SYSTEM
□ ■ ■

bactericidal, tonic > arrests bleeding

SKIN, MUSCLES and BODY TISSUES
■ □ ■ ■

antiseptic, parasiticide > arthritis, boils, cuts, fleas, muscular aches and pains, rheumatism, ringworm, scabies, wounds

RESPIRATORY SYSTEM
■ □ ■ ■

expectorant > bronchitis, catarrh, whooping cough

DIGESTIVE SYSTEM

URINARY SYSTEM
■ □ ■ ■

diuretic > cystitis, urethritis

REPRODUCTIVE SYSTEM
■

mucolytic > leucorrhoea

BOTANICAL FAMILY

Pinaceae : this family is generally highly antiseptic and aids respiratory problems.

Tree: distilled oleoresin from wood chips : warm soothing aroma : middle note.
Used by Galen and Hippocrates. Used in China both internally and externally for hundreds of years. Most commonly used now for paint and stain remover but still used extensively in many ointments and lotions for aches and pains.

Chemical constituents may include:

■ bornyl acetate

■ borneol, pinocarveol, terpineol, fenchol

□ α-pinene, β-pinene

■ methyl chavicol (estragole)

PINE LONGLEAF WOOD
Pinus palustris

☐ ketones	1.0%
☐ remainder	2.9%
☐ oxides	0.1%
☐ monoterpenes	8.0%
■ alcohols	80.0%
■ phenols,phe. ethers	8.0%

Stimulating   Balancing   Relaxing

BODY SYSTEMS

PROPERTIES > USES

NERVOUS SYSTEM
☐☐■■■

analgesic, stimulant >

ENDOCRINE SYSTEM

CIRCULATION AND IMMUNE SYSTEM
☐☐☐■■

bactericidal, decongestant > stimulates circulation

SKIN, MUSCLES and BODY TISSUES
☐☐■■■

antiseptic, insecticide > arthritis, lumbago, rheumatism

RESPIRATORY SYSTEM
☐☐■■■

expectorant > asthma, bronchitis, catarrh, sinusitis

DIGESTIVE SYSTEM

URINARY SYSTEM

REPRODUCTIVE SYSTEM

BOTANICAL FAMILY

Pinaceae : this family is generally highly antiseptic and aids respiratory problems.

Tree: distilled heartwood : sweet soothing pine aroma : middle note.
Pine sawdust poultices have been used very successfully for rheumatism, hard cancerous deposits and lumbago.

Chemical constituents may include:

☐ fenchone

■ terpineol, fenchol, borneol

☐ α-pinene, β-pinene

■ methyl chavicol (estragole)

PINE SCOTCH
Pinus sylvestris

■	esters	5.0%
■	aliphatic aldehydes	yes
□	ketones	yes
■	sesquiterpenes	5.0%
□	remainder	15.0%
□	oxides	yes
□	acids	yes
■	aromatic aldehydes	yes
■	monoterpenes	70.0%
■	alcohols	5.0%
■	phenols,phe. ethers	yes

Stimulating   Balancing   Relaxing

BODY SYSTEMS

NERVOUS SYSTEM
■ ■ ■ □ ■ ■ ■ ■

ENDOCRINE SYSTEM
■ ■ ■ ■ ■

CIRCULATION AND IMMUNE SYSTEM
■ ■ □ ■ ■ ■

SKIN, MUSCLES and BODY TISSUES
■ ■ ■ ■ ■ ■ ■

RESPIRATORY SYSTEM
■ ■ ■ ■ □ ■ ■ ■

DIGESTIVE SYSTEM
■ ■ ■ ■ □ ■ ■ ■

URINARY SYSTEM
■ ■ ■ ■ □ ■ ■ ■

REPRODUCTIVE SYSTEM
■ ■ ■ ■ ■ ■ ■

CAUTIONS
BOTANICAL FAMILY

PROPERTIES > USES

analgesic, aphrodisiac, stimulant, tonic > frigidity, impotence, multiple sclerosis

cortisone like, hormone like, temperature balancing > adrenal glands

bactericidal, decongestant, raises blood pressure > lymph system

antifungal, antiinflammatory, antiseptic > allergies, arthritis, eczema, muscular aches and pains, psoriasis

expectorant > asthma, excellent for bronchitis, sinusitis

stimulates secretions > diabetes, gall stones, gastric, hepatitis, indigestion

diuretic > cystitis

decongestant > fallopian tubes, ovaries, stimulates egg and sperm production, uterus

Use with care check sensitive skin for irritation.

Pinaceae : this family is generally highly antiseptic and aids respiratory problems.

Tree: distilled dry needles : fresh forest aroma : middle note.
It is acknowledged that the pine forests produce a healing enviroment due to the evaporation of the essential oil from the pine needles.
Chemical constituents may include:

■ bornyl acetate, terpinyl acetate

■ citronellal, citral

□ cryptone

■ caryophyllene, cadinene, copaene, guaiene, farnesene

■ cuminaldehyde, anisaldehyde

■ α-pinene, β-pinene, limonene, Δ^3-carene, camphene, phellandrene, dipentene, terpinenes, myrcene, sabinene

■ borneol, terpinen-4-ol, cadinol

RAVENSARA AROMATIC
Ravensara aromatica

■ esters	yes
■ sesquiterpenes	yes
□ remainder	18.0%
□ oxides	60.0%
■ monoterpenes	14.0%
■ alcohols	8.0%

Stimulating   Balancing   Relaxing

BODY SYSTEMS	PROPERTIES > USES
NERVOUS SYSTEM ■■□■■	tonic > dendritis, insomnia
ENDOCRINE SYSTEM □■■	tonic > glandular fever
CIRCULATION AND IMMUNE SYSTEM ■■■	antiviral, bactericidal >
SKIN, MUSCLES and BODY TISSUES ■■■■	antifungal, antiseptic > chicken pox, herpes, muscle aches and pains
RESPIRATORY SYSTEM ■■□■■	expectorant > bronchitis, flu, sinusitis, whooping cough
DIGESTIVE SYSTEM ■■□■■	stimulates secretions > enteritis, gastric, liver
URINARY SYSTEM	
REPRODUCTIVE SYSTEM	

BOTANICAL FAMILY   Lauraceae : this family is usually powerful and stimulating.

Shrub: distilled foliage : clear aroma : middle note.
Relaxing to system when massaged over the vertebral column.

Chemical constituents may include:

■ terpinyl acetate

■ β-caryophyllene

□ 1.8-cineole

■ α-pinene, β-pinene, sabinene

■ α-terpineol, terpinen-4-ol

ROSE OTTO
Rosa damascena

■	esters	4.0%
■	aliphatic aldehydes	0.5%
▩	ketones	yes
■	sesquiterpenes	1.0%
□	remainder	12.8%
□	oxides	0.3%
▨	monoterpenes	20.0%
■	alcohols	60.0%
■	phenols,phe. ethers	1.4%

Stimulating   Balancing   Relaxing

BODY SYSTEMS

NERVOUS SYSTEM
■■■■□■■■

ENDOCRINE SYSTEM
■■■■

CIRCULATION AND IMMUNE SYSTEM
■■■■■

SKIN, MUSCLES and BODY TISSUES
■■■■□■■

RESPIRATORY SYSTEM
■■■■■■■

DIGESTIVE SYSTEM
□□■■■

URINARY SYSTEM
□□■■■

REPRODUCTIVE SYSTEM
■■□■■■

PROPERTIES > USES

aphrodisiac, antispasmodic, balancing, calming, cheering, sedative, tonic > jealousy, increases confidence, Raynaud's disease

regulates, hormone like, stimulates pituarity gland > releases dopamine

bactericidal, decongestant, purifies > stops bleeding, broken veins, tones capillaries, conjunctivitis

antiinflammatory, antiseptic > gingivitis, skin infections, wounds

bactericidal > asthma, bronchitis, coughs, TB

tonic > increases bile production, jaundice, liver, spleen

diuretic >

emmenagogue > frigidity, impotence, pmt

BOTANICAL FAMILY   Rosaceae.

Shrub: distilled petals : sweet heavenly flowery aroma : base note.
Symbol of love and purity. Women's oil to calm and relieve tension and feelings of inadequacy. Scent due to damascenone (only 0.14%)(25).

Chemical constituents may include:

- ■ citronellyl acetate, geranyl acetate, neryl acetate
- ■ neral
- ■ caryophyllene
- □ damascenone

- □ rose oxide
- ■ stearoptene, camphene, myrcene, cymene, pinenes, ocimene
- ■ citronellol, geraniol, farnesol, nerol, linalool, phenylethyl alcohol
- ■ methyl eugenol

ROSEMARY
Rosmarinus officinalis

■ esters	1.0%
■ ketones	25.0%
■ sesquiterpenes	3.0%
☐ remainder	8.0%
☐ oxides	30.0%
■ monoterpenes	30.0%
■ alcohols	3.0%

Stimulating   Balancing   Relaxing

BODY SYSTEMS

NERVOUS SYSTEM
■■■□□■

ENDOCRINE SYSTEM
□□■■

CIRCULATION AND IMMUNE SYSTEM
■■■■

SKIN, MUSCLES and BODY TISSUES
■■■□□■

RESPIRATORY SYSTEM
■■■□□■

DIGESTIVE SYSTEM
■■■□□■

URINARY SYSTEM
■■■□□■

REPRODUCTIVE SYSTEM
■■■□□■

CAUTIONS

BOTANICAL FAMILY

PROPERTIES > USES

analgesic, antispasmodic, stimulant, stimulates memory > bedwetting, general fatigue, depression, migraine, Raynaud's disease

stimulates secretions > stimulates central nervous system and bile production

antiviral, astringent, bactericidal, low/high dose lowers/raises blood pressure > arteriosclerosis, circulation, heart

antifungal, antiinflammatory, antiseptic > dissolves swellings and boils, otitis, rheumatism, whooping cough

expectorant, decongestant, mucolytic, stimulant > catarrh, flu

stimulant > constipation, cirrhosis, diarrhoea, flatulence, gall bladder, hepatitis

diuretic > cystitis

emmenagogue > amenorrhoea, candida, scanty periods

Do not use if epilepsy is suspected (26).

Lamiaceae.

Herb: distilled flowering stalks : strong herbal aroma : middle note.
Name means seadew - Greeks and Romans considered it to be a sacred plant bringing peace and comfort. Can help temporary paralysis and speech problems. Smooth muscle relaxant(27).

Chemical constituents may include:

■ bornyl acetate, fenchyl acetate

☐ camphor, carvone, thujone, octanone

■ caryophyllene, humulene

☐ 1.8-cineole, caryophyllene oxide

■ α-pinene, β-pinene, camphene, myrcene, limonene, p-cymene

■ terpineol, linalool, borneol, terpinen-4-ol

ROSEWOOD
Aniba rosaeodora

■	aliphatic aldehydes	yes
◫	ketones	yes
☐	remainder	10.0%
☐	oxides	yes
◪	monoterpenes	yes
■	alcohols	90.0%

Stimulating   Balancing   Relaxing

BODY SYSTEMS

NERVOUS SYSTEM
■ ☐ ☐ ■ ■

ENDOCRINE SYSTEM

CIRCULATION AND IMMUNE SYSTEM
■ ☐ ☐ ■

SKIN, MUSCLES and BODY TISSUES
■ ☐ ☐ ■ ■

RESPIRATORY SYSTEM
■ ☐ ☐ ■ ■

DIGESTIVE SYSTEM

URINARY SYSTEM

REPRODUCTIVE SYSTEM
■ ☐ ■

PROPERTIES > USES

analgesic, aphrodisiac, stimulant, tonic > clears mind, depression

antiviral, bactericidal, immune system tonic > chronic conditions

antifungal, antiseptic, deodorant, insecticide > skin tonic and healer

antiseptic > bronchopneumonia, ticklish coughs

antifungal > candida

BOTANICAL FAMILY

Lauraceae : the gentle member of this family which is generally powerful and stimulating.

Tree: distilled heartwood : sweet floral woody aroma : middle note.
Brazilian exploitation of the forests to produce oil has now been restricted and replanting programmes are in place.

Chemical constituents may include:

■ citronellal

☐ 1.8-cineole, linalool oxide

◪ α-terpinene, limonene, β-pinene

■ linalool, geraniol, nerol, α-terpineol

SAGE COMMON
Salvia officinalis

esters	2.5%
aliphatic aldehydes	yes
ketones	35.0%
sesquiterpenes	12.0%
lactones and coumarins	yes
remainder	1.0%
oxides	8.0%
aromatic aldehydes	10.0%
monoterpenes	20.0%
alcohols	8.0%
phenols,phe. ethers	3.5%

Stimulating   Balancing   Relaxing

BODY SYSTEMS

NERVOUS SYSTEM
■■■■■□■■■■

ENDOCRINE SYSTEM
□■

CIRCULATION AND IMMUNE SYSTEM
■■■■■□■■■■

SKIN, MUSCLES and BODY TISSUES
■■■■■□■■■■

RESPIRATORY SYSTEM
■■■■■□■■■■

DIGESTIVE SYSTEM
□□■■■

URINARY SYSTEM
□□■■■

REPRODUCTIVE SYSTEM
■■■■■□■■■■

CAUTIONS

BOTANICAL FAMILY

PROPERTIES > USES

analgesic, antispasmodic, tonic > eases trembling, meningitis, neuritis, palsy

stops milk production, stimulates secretions > bile

antiviral, bactericidal, decongestant, purifies, raises blood pressure, tonic > balances circulation

antifungal, antiseptic > cellulite, malignancies, oedema, psoriasis, rheumatoid arthritis, toothache, ulcers, wounds
expectorant, mucolytic > bronchitis, catarrh, flu

stimulant, tonic > bile, liver, pancreas

diuretic >

abortive, emmenagogue > candida, genital herpes, hot flushes, leucorrhoea, thrush

Avoid in pregnancy. Do not use with young children or epileptics. Not recommended by some practitioners.
Lamiaceae.

Herb: distilled flowering herb : sharp herbal aroma : top note.
Hailed as a miracle plant by the Romans - 'salvare' means to heal, to save. Used as a nerve tonic through the middle ages.

Chemical constituents may include:

■ bornyl acetate, linalyl acetate

■ hexanal

□ α-thujone, β-thujone, camphor, fenchone

■ caryophyllene, humulene, cadinene

□ 1.8-cineole, caryophyllene oxide

■ α-pinene, β-pinene, phellandrene, camphene, myrcene, limonene, p-cymene
borneol, viridiflorol, linalool, terpinen-4-ol

■ methyl chavicol (estragole), thymol

SAGE SPANISH
Salvia lavendulaefolia

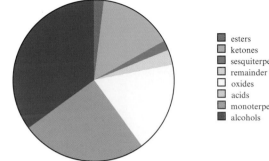

■	esters	2.0%
□	ketones	15.0%
■	sesquiterpenes	2.0%
□	remainder	3.0%
□	oxides	18.0%
■	acids	yes
■	monoterpenes	25.0%
■	alcohols	35.0%

Stimulating   Balancing   Relaxing

BODY SYSTEMS

NERVOUS SYSTEM
■■■□■■

ENDOCRINE SYSTEM
■■■■

CIRCULATION AND IMMUNE SYSTEM
■■□■■

SKIN, MUSCLES and BODY TISSUES
■■■□■■■

RESPIRATORY SYSTEM
■■□■■

DIGESTIVE SYSTEM
■■□■■

URINARY SYSTEM

REPRODUCTIVE SYSTEM
■■■□■■

CAUTIONS

BOTANICAL FAMILY

PROPERTIES > USES

antispasmodic, tonic > headaches, nervous exhaustion, neuralgia

lowers fever, regulates sebum production, reduces sweating > stimulates liver and adrenal cortex

astringent, lowers blood pressure > circulation, purifies blood

antiinflammatory, antiseptic > acne, arthritis, eczema, fluid retention, gingivitis, hair loss, rheumatism, wounds

decongestant, expectorant > asthma, catarrh, coughs, flu, rhinitis, sinusitis

stimulant > congested liver, jaundice

emmenagogue > amenorrhoea, painful periods

Avoid in pregnancy. Use in moderation.

Lamiaceae.

Herb: distilled flowering herb : sage like lavender aroma : top note.
In Spain considered a 'cure all'. Some chemotypes have much higher percentages of camphor present hence the need for caution.

Chemical constituents may include:

■ linalyl acetate, bornyl acetate, sabinyl acetate, terpinyl acetate

■ camphor

■ caryophyllene, humulene, bergaptene

□ 1.8-cineole

■ α-pinene, β-pinene, sabinene, myrcene, camphene, limonene, p-cymene

■ linalool, α-terpineol, borneol, sabinol, geraniol

SANDALWOOD
Santalum album

▦ aliphatic aldehydes	yes
☐ ketones	yes
▦ sesquiterpenes	10.0%
☐ lactones and coumarins	yes
☐ remainder	7.5%
☐ acids	2.5%
☐ monoterpenes	yes
■ alcohols	80.0%
■ phenols,phe. ethers	yes

Stimulating   Balancing   Relaxing

BODY SYSTEMS	PROPERTIES > USES
NERVOUS SYSTEM ■■■■■	aphrodisiac, calming, sedative, tonic > bereavement, impotence, neuralgia, sciatica
ENDOCRINE SYSTEM ■■	promotes vaginal secretions >
CIRCULATION AND IMMUNE SYSTEM ■■■■■	astringent, bactericidal, decongestant > heart regulation, varicose veins
SKIN, MUSCLES and BODY TISSUES ■■■■■■	antiinflammatory, antiseptic > aging skin, dry ezcema, itching, haemorrhoids, lumbago
RESPIRATORY SYSTEM ■■■■■■	calming > catarrh, eases coughs
DIGESTIVE SYSTEM ■■■	calming > diarrhoea
URINARY SYSTEM ■■■■	diuretic > cystitis, kidney
REPRODUCTIVE SYSTEM ■■■■■	antiseptic > gonorrhoea

BOTANICAL FAMILY   Santalaceae.

Tree: distilled heartwood : musty lingering aroma : base note.
Brings peaceful feelings. Comfort to the dying. Used in incenses and meditation.

Chemical constituents may include:

☐ santalone

■ santalenes, curcumenes, farnesene

☐ limonene

☐ nortricycloekasantalic acid

■ santalols, tricycloekasantalol, borneol

SAVORY SUMMER
Satureja hortensis

☐	ketones	yes
☐	sesquiterpenes	3.5%
☐	remainder	21.5%
☐	oxides	yes
☐	acids	yes
☐	aromatic aldehydes	yes
☐	monoterpenes	34.0%
☐	alcohols	1.0%
■	phenols,phe. ethers	40.0%

Stimulating   Balancing   Relaxing

BODY SYSTEMS	PROPERTIES > USES
NERVOUS SYSTEM ■ ■ ☐ ■ ■ ■ ■	aphrodisiac, general tonic >
ENDOCRINE SYSTEM ■ ■	stimulates secretions > bile
CIRCULATION AND IMMUNE SYSTEM ■ ☐ ■ ■ ■ ■	antiviral, astringent, strongly bactericidal, tonic > cardiac
SKIN, MUSCLES and BODY TISSUES ■ ■ ☐ ■ ■ ■ ■	antifungal, air antiseptic, irritant, parasiticide, vulnerary > any infected location
RESPIRATORY SYSTEM ■ ■ ■ ☐ ■ ■ ■ ■	expectorant > mucous membrane irritant
DIGESTIVE SYSTEM ■ ■ ☐ ■ ■ ■	stimulant > liver, facilitates elimination, flatulence
URINARY SYSTEM	
REPRODUCTIVE SYSTEM ☐ ■ ■ ■	sexual tonic >

CAUTIONS	Avoid during pregnancy. Not recommended for use by some practitioners due to high phenol content. Do not use directly onto skin.
BOTANICAL FAMILY	Lamiaceae.

Herb: distilled whole dried herb : strong thyme like aroma : top note.
Closely related to the thymes. Popular for cookery, peppery flavour. Therapeutic tea for digestion, respiratory and menstrual problems.

Chemical constituents may include:

- ☐ camphor
- ■ β-caryophyllene, bisabolene, cadinene
- ☐ damascenone
- ☐ 1.8-cineole
- ■ piperonal
- ☐ α-terpinene, γ-terpinene, p-cymene, myrcene, pinenes, limonene, phellandrene
- ■ linalool, borneol, terpineol, terpinen-4-ol
- ■ thymol, eugenol, carvacrol

SAVORY WINTER
Satureja montana

■ esters	2.0%
□ ketones	yes
■ sesquiterpenes	2.0%
□ remainder	5.0%
□ oxides	1.0%
□ acids	yes
■ monoterpenes	30.0%
■ alcohols	20.0%
■ phenols,phe. ethers	40.0%

Stimulating   Balancing   Relaxing

BODY SYSTEMS

PROPERTIES > USES

NERVOUS SYSTEM
■■■□■■■

general tonic, mental stimulant, neurotonic > depression, nervous exhaustion

ENDOCRINE SYSTEM

CIRCULATION AND IMMUNE SYSTEM
■■□■■■

antiviral, strongly bactericidal, raises blood pressure, immune system tonic > circulation

SKIN, MUSCLES and BODY TISSUES
■■■■□□■■■

antifungal, strongly antiseptic, irritant > abscesses, fungal infection of mouth, impetigo, rheumatoid arthritis

RESPIRATORY SYSTEM
■■□■■■

bactericidal > bronchitis, coughs, malaria, TB

DIGESTIVE SYSTEM
■■■□■■■

bactericidal > colic, colitis, diarrhoea, enteritis, flatulence, intestinal spasm

URINARY SYSTEM
■■■□■■■

diuretic > cystitis, prostate, renal TB

REPRODUCTIVE SYSTEM
■■■

antifungal > candida

CAUTIONS

Avoid in pregnancy. Not recommended for use by some practitioners due to its high phenol content. Do not use directly onto skin.

BOTANICAL FAMILY

Lamiaceae.

Herb: distilled whole dried herb : herby medicinal aroma : top note.
Highly antiseptic properties.

Chemical constituents may include:
- ■ linalyl acetate, terpinyl acetate, geranyl acetate
- □ camphor
- ■ β-caryophyllene, humulene
- □ damascenone

- □ 1.8-cineole, caryophyllene oxide
- ■ α-terpinene,γ-terpinene, p-cymene, α-pinene, β-pinene, limonene
- ■ linalool, borneol, α-terpineol, thujanols
- ■ carvacrol, thymol, eugenol

SPRUCE CANADIAN BLACK
Picea mariana nigra

■	esters	35.0%
■	ketones	1.0%
■	sesquiterpenes	1.0%
☐	remainder	5.5%
■	monoterpenes	55.0%
■	alcohols	2.5%

Stimulating   Balancing   Relaxing

BODY SYSTEMS	PROPERTIES > USES
NERVOUS SYSTEM ■ ■ ■ ■	antispasmodic, tonic > revitalising
ENDOCRINE SYSTEM ☐ ■	cortisone like, hormone like > overactive thyroid, ovaries, thymus gland
CIRCULATION AND IMMUNE SYSTEM ■ ■ ■	bactericidal, immune system tonic >
SKIN, MUSCLES and BODY TISSUES ■ ■ ■ ■ ■	antifungal, antiinflammatory, air antiseptic, tonic > acne, eczema, rheumatism
RESPIRATORY SYSTEM ■ ■ ■ ■ ■	bactericidal > bronchitis
DIGESTIVE SYSTEM	
URINARY SYSTEM	
REPRODUCTIVE SYSTEM ■ ☐ ■	antifungal > candida

BOTANICAL FAMILY   Pinaceae : this family is generally highly antiseptic and aids respiratory problems.

Tree: distilled young branches and leaves : pleasant pine needle aroma : middle note. Often added to pine and cedar oils.

Chemical constituents may include:

- ■ bornyl acetate
- ☐ camphor
- ■ longifolene, longicyclene, cadinene
- ■ tricyclene, α-pinene, Δ^3-carene, camphene
- ■ borneol, longiborneol

SPRUCE HEMLOCK
Tsuga canadensis

■	esters	45.0%
■	aliphatic aldehydes	yes
□	ketones	2.5%
■	sesquiterpenes	yes
□	remainder	2.5%
■	monoterpenes	45.0%
■	alcohols	5.0%

Stimulating   Balancing   Relaxing

BODY SYSTEMS

NERVOUS SYSTEM
■ ■ ■ ■ ■   calming, stimulant > anxiety, stress

ENDOCRINE SYSTEM

CIRCULATION AND IMMUNE SYSTEM   bactericidal, stems bleeding, lymph system tonic >
■ ■ ■ ■   lymph circulation

SKIN, MUSCLES and BODY TISSUES   antiseptic > aches and pains, rheumatism
■ ■ ■ ■ ■

RESPIRATORY SYSTEM   expectorant > asthma, bronchitis, coughs, weakness
■ ■ ■ ■ ■

DIGESTIVE SYSTEM

URINARY SYSTEM   diuretic >
■ ■ ■

REPRODUCTIVE SYSTEM

BOTANICAL FAMILY   Pinaceae : this family is generally highly antiseptic and
                                 aids respiratory problems.

Tree: distilled needles and twigs : fresh fruity sweet aroma : middle note.
Widely used for veterinary linaments and for room sprays.

Chemical constituents may include:

■ bornyl acetate   □ pinenes, limonene, tricyclene, camphene,
                            myrcene, phellandrene, dipentene
□ thujone
                          ■ borneol
■ cadinene

TAGETES
Tagetes glandulifera

■ aliphatic aldehydes	yes
☐ ketones	50.0%
■ lactones and coumarins	yes
☐ remainder	15.0%
☐ acids	yes
■ aromatic aldehydes	yes
■ monoterpenes	35.0%
■ alcohols	yes

Stimulating   Balancing   Relaxing

BODY SYSTEMS	PROPERTIES > USES
NERVOUS SYSTEM ■ ■ ■ ■ ■	antispasmodic, sedative > clears mind, firmer hold on emotions, relieves tension, sharpens senses
ENDOCRINE SYSTEM	
CIRCULATION AND IMMUNE SYSTEM ■ ■ ■ ■ ■	bactericidal, lowers blood pressure >
SKIN, MUSCLES and BODY TISSUES ■ ■ ■ ■ ■ ■	antifungal, antiinflammatory, antiseptic, cell generator, insectiticide > athlete's foot, bunions, callouses, corns, flies, ear infections, maggots, mosquitoes
RESPIRATORY SYSTEM ■ ■ ■ ■	decongestant > affinity to respiratory system, bronchial dilator, coughs
DIGESTIVE SYSTEM	
URINARY SYSTEM	
REPRODUCTIVE SYSTEM ■	emmenagogue >
CAUTIONS	Powerful oil use with care, check for skin irritation.
BOTANICAL FAMILY	Compositae : this family is generally soothing especially for the skin and digestion.

Plant: distilled after the full flowering stage : strong marigold aroma : top note.
Often planted among vegetables to deter pests. Used extensively in french perfumes.

Chemical constituents may include:

- ■ citral
- ■ tagetone, tagetenones, carvone
- ☐ valeric acid

- ■ salicylaldehyde
- ■ pinenes, limonene, ocimene, myrcene, camphene
- ■ linalool

81

TARRAGON
Artemisia dracunculus

ketones		yes
lactones and coumarins		0.1%
remainder		29.9%
oxides		yes
monoterpenes		yes
alcohols		yes
phenols,phe. ethers		70.0%

Stimulating Balancing Relaxing

BODY SYSTEMS

NERVOUS SYSTEM

ENDOCRINE SYSTEM

CIRCULATION AND IMMUNE SYSTEM

SKIN, MUSCLES and BODY TISSUES

RESPIRATORY SYSTEM

DIGESTIVE SYSTEM

URINARY SYSTEM

REPRODUCTIVE SYSTEM

CAUTIONS

BOTANICAL FAMILY

PROPERTIES > USES

antispasmodic, hypnotic, neuromuscular tonic, stimulant > allergies, neuralgia, pmt, sciatica

balances menstrual cycle, stimulates secretion > bile

antiviral, bactericidal, decongestant, purifies > chronic conditions

antiinflammatory, antiseptic > arthritis (clears uric acid), rheumatism, weeping wounds

decongestant > hiccoughs

stimulates appetite > anorexia, bile secretion, digestion heavy fats, inflamed intestines, laxative, spasms, worms
diuretic > cleanses kidneys

emmenagogue > amenorrhoea, menstrual, painful periods, pmt

Avoid in pregnancy, use with care due to large amount of phenols present.

Compositae : this family is generally soothing especially for the skin and digestion.

Herb: distilled leaves : spicy aniseed like aroma : top note.
Very popular culinary herb rich in vitamins A and C. Has been used to treat snake and dog bites.

Chemical constituents may include:

- thujone
- aesculetin, methyl oxycoumarin, herniarine
- 1.8-cineole
- ocimene, phellandrene
- nerol
- methyl chavicol (estragole), anethole

82

TEATREE
Melaleuca alternifolia

■ sesquiterpenes	6.0%
□ remainder	1.0%
□ oxides	7.0%
□ acids	yes
■ monoterpenes	41.0%
■ alcohols	45.0%

Stimulating   Balancing   Relaxing

BODY SYSTEMS	PROPERTIES > USES
NERVOUS SYSTEM ■ □□■	analgesic, neurotonic > depression, hysteria, shock
ENDOCRINE SYSTEM ■ □	causes sweating >
CIRCULATION AND IMMUNE SYSTEM ■ ■ □□■	antiviral, strongly bactericidal, decongestant, immune system tonic, heart tonic > varicose veins
SKIN, MUSCLES AND BODY TISSUES ■ ■ □□□■	antifungal, antiinflammatory, strongly antiseptic, parasiticide > athlete's foot, bites, boils, burns, radiography burns, cold sores, itching, mouth ulcers, ringworm, spots, sweaty feet, wounds
RESPIRATORY SYSTEM ■ □■■	bactericidal > asthma, bronchitis, catarrh, TB, whooping cough
DIGESTIVE SYSTEM ■ ■■	antiseptic > haemorrhoids, mouth infections
URINARY SYSTEM ■ ■■	bactericidal > cystitis
REPRODUCTIVE SYSTEM □■■	antifungal > candida, congested ovaries, thrush
BOTANICAL FAMILY	Myrtaceae : this family is generally stimulating and good for the respiratory system.

Shrub: distilled leaves : pungent sanitary aroma : top note.
Extensively used in aboriginal medicine, wide spread current use including surgical and dental practices. Strong antifungal agent(14).

Chemical constituents may include:

■ aromadendrene, viridiflorene, cadinene, caryophyllene

□ 1.8-cineole, 1.4-cineole

■ α-pinene, α-terpinene, γ-terpinene p-cymene, limonene, terpinolene, myrcene

■ terpinen-4-ol, α-terpineol, globulol, viridiflorol

THUJA WHITE CEDAR
Thuja occidentalis

■	esters	5.0%
□	ketones	70.0%
■	sesquiterpenes	yes
□	remainder	6.0%
□	acids	yes
■	monoterpenes	14.0%
■	alcohols	5.0%

Stimulating   Balancing   Relaxing

BODY SYSTEMS	PROPERTIES > USES
NERVOUS SYSTEM □ ■	stimulant >
ENDOCRINE SYSTEM	
CIRCULATION AND IMMUNE SYSTEM □ □ ■	astringent, heart tonic >
SKIN, MUSCLES and BODY TISSUES ■ ■ ■ □ □ ■	stimulant > insect repellent, rheumatism, warts
RESPIRATORY SYSTEM □ □	expectorant >
DIGESTIVE SYSTEM □	parasiticide, vermifuge > poison
URINARY SYSTEM □ □ ■	diuretic >
REPRODUCTIVE SYSTEM □ □ ■	abortive, stimulant >
CAUTIONS	Not recommended for use except in exceptional circumstances(28).
BOTANICAL FAMILY	Cupressaceae : this family generally aids nervous tension, rheumatism and cellulite.

Tree: distilled leaves twigs and bark : sharp camphor like aroma : top note.
Used as incense by ancient civilisations. Twigs are currently in the British Herbal Pharmacoepia for cardiac weakness, bronchitis and warts.

Chemical constituents may include:

■ bornyl acetate

□ thujone, camphor, fenchone, piperitone, isothujone

■ pinene, sabinene

■ terpinen-4-ol, occidentalol, occidol

84

THYME COMMON RED or WHITE
Thymus vulgaris thymoliferum

■ esters	2.0%
■ ketones	9.0%
■ sesquiterpenes	1.5%
□ remainder	1.5%
□ oxides	4.0%
■ acids	yes
■ monoterpenes	25.0%
■ alcohols	17.0%
■ phenols,phe. ethers	40.0%

Stimulating   Balancing   Relaxing

BODY SYSTEMS	PROPERTIES > USES
NERVOUS SYSTEM ■■■□■■■	antispasmodic, general and neurotonic, mental sexual tonic, stimulant > depression, stress
ENDOCRINE SYSTEM □□■■■	causes sweating > stimulates white corpuscles
CIRCULATION AND IMMUNE SYSTEM ■■□■■■	bactericidal, raises blood pressure, capillary stimulant > anaemia, circulation
SKIN, MUSCLES and BODY TISSUES ■■■□□□■■	antioxidant, antiseptic, parasiticide > acne, arthritis, boils, carbuncles, hair loss, rheumatism, wounds
RESPIRATORY SYSTEM ■■■□■■	expectorant > anxiety, asthma, bronchial secretions
DIGESTIVE SYSTEM ■■■□■■	stimulant > flatulence, sluggish digestion, worms
URINARY SYSTEM ■■■□■■	diuretic > cystitis
REPRODUCTIVE SYSTEM □□■■	mucolytic > assists childbirth helps to expel afterbirth, leucorrhoea
CAUTIONS	Avoid in cases of pregnancy or high blood pressure.
BOTANICAL FAMILY	Lamiaceae.

Herb: distilled fresh or part dried leaves and flowering tops : strong herby aroma : top note. Composition of thyme oils is complex to identify. Strongly bactericidal(13). Red Thyme and White Thyme have high phenol content as shown above. White Thyme is a refined distillation of Red Thyme. Sweet Thyme is a very different oil and is shown on page 86.

Chemical constituents may include:

■ linalyl acetate, terpinyl acetate

□ camphor, thujone

■ β-caryophyllene

□ 1.8-cineole, linalool oxide

■ p-cymene, γ-terpinene, α-pinene, camphene, myrcene, limonene, terpinolene

■ borneol, linalool, terpinen-4-ol

■ thymol, carvacrol

THYME COMMON SWEET
Thymus vulgaris linaloliferum or geranioliferum

esters	40.0%	
ketones	yes	
sesquiterpenes	yes	
remainder	15.0%	
oxides	yes	
acids	yes	
monoterpenes	10.0%	
alcohols	35.0%	
phenols,phe. ethers	yes	

Stimulating   Balancing   Relaxing

BODY SYSTEMS	PROPERTIES > USES
NERVOUS SYSTEM ■■■□■■■	antispasmodic > fatigue
ENDOCRINE SYSTEM ■	stimulates secretions > bile
CIRCULATION AND IMMUNE SYSTEM ■■■□■■■	antiviral > heart stimulant
SKIN, MUSCLES and BODY TISSUES ■■■□■■■■	antioxidant, antifungal, antiinflammatory, antiseptic > acne, dry and wet eczema, muscular rheumatism, psoriasis, verrucas
RESPIRATORY SYSTEM ■■■□■■■	antiseptic > bronchitis, bronchial spasm, sinusitis, sore throat, tonsillitis, TB
DIGESTIVE SYSTEM ■■■□■■■	antiviral > colitis, diarrhoea, liver, viral enteritis
URINARY SYSTEM ■■■□■■■	antiseptic > cystitis, urethritis
REPRODUCTIVE SYSTEM ■■■□■■■	antifungal, uterine tonic > assists childbirth, candida, vaginitis

BOTANICAL FAMILY   Lamiaceae.

Herb: distilled fresh or part dried leaves and flowering tops : sweet lemon aroma : top note.
Much safer to use than thymus vulgaris thymoliferum (red or white thyme).

Chemical constituents may include:

■ linalyl acetate, geranyl acetate   ■ linalool or geraniol

THYME MOROCCAN
Thymus satureioides

■ esters	4.0%
■ aliphatic aldehydes	yes
□ ketones	2.0%
■ sesquiterpenes	5.0%
□ remainder	2.0%
□ oxides	2.0%
□ acids	yes
■ monoterpenes	15.0%
■ alcohols	30.0%
■ phenols,phe. ethers	40.0%

Stimulating   Balancing   Relaxing

BODY SYSTEMS	PROPERTIES > USES
NERVOUS SYSTEM ■■■■□□■■	sexual tonic, stimulant, neurotonic > debility, general fatigue
ENDOCRINE SYSTEM □■	stimulates secretions > gall bladder, gastric, liver
CIRCULATION AND IMMUNE SYSTEM ■□□■■	bactericidal, immune system tonic >
SKIN, MUSCLES and BODY TISSUES ■■■■□□□■■	antiinflammatory, antiseptic, possible irritant > acne, arthritis, chronic sinusitis, tonsillitis
RESPIRATORY SYSTEM ■■□■■	bactericidal > TB
DIGESTIVE SYSTEM □■	secretions > gall bladder, gall stones, liver
URINARY SYSTEM ■■■□□■■	bactericidal > cystitis
REPRODUCTIVE SYSTEM □■■	uterine tonic >

BOTANICAL FAMILY   Lamiaceae.

Herb: distilled flowering tops : herby aroma : top note.
Similar properties to thymus vulgaris thymoliferum (red or white thyme).

Chemical constituents may include:

■ bornyl acetate, linalyl acetate

■ dihydrocarvone, verbenone, camphor

■ caryophyllene, cadinene, copaene, bourbonene, humulene

□ 1.8-cineole, caryophyllene oxide, linalool oxide

■ α-pinene, γ-terpinene, p-cymene, camphene

■ borneol, terpineol, terpinen-4-ol, linalool

■ methyl chavicol (estragole), thymol, carvacrol

VETIVER
Vetiveria zizanioides

■ esters		yes
□ ketones		15.0%
■ sesquiterpenes		yes
□ remainder		45.0%
□ acids		yes
■ alcohols		40.0%

Stimulating   Balancing   Relaxing

BODY SYSTEMS   **PROPERTIES > USES**

NERVOUS SYSTEM
■ ■ ■ ■
aphrodisiac, calming, sedative, tonic > dentist's visit, over sensitivity, protective shield, stress, tension

ENDOCRINE SYSTEM
□ □ □ ■
stimulant to glands > promotes bleeding, promotes pancreas secretions

CIRCULATION AND IMMUNE SYSTEM
□ □ ■
immune system tonic, stimulates blood flow > coronary arteries, veins

SKIN, MUSCLES and BODY TISSUES
■ □ □ □ ■
antiseptic > aches and pains, acne, arthritis, rheumatism

RESPIRATORY SYSTEM

DIGESTIVE SYSTEM
□ ■
stimulant > congested liver, pancreas

URINARY SYSTEM

REPRODUCTIVE SYSTEM
□ □ ■
emmenagogue > amenorrhoea, scanty periods

BOTANICAL FAMILY   Gramineae.

Grass: distilled roots : earthy woody aroma : base note.
Known as the oil of tranquillity. The grass is called 'kuskus' and is used to make awnings, sunshades and blinds. Beautiful aroma when dampened.

Chemical constituents may include:

■ vetiverol acetate

□ furfural

□ vetiverone

□ vetivenic acid, benzoic acid, palmitic acid

■ vetivene, vetivazulene

■ vetiverol

YARROW
Achillea millefolium

esters	2.0%
ketones	9.0%
sesquiterpenes	45.0%
lactones and coumarins	yes
remainder	2.0%
oxides	7.0%
acids	yes
monoterpenes	28.0%
alcohols	7.0%
phenols,phe. ethers	yes

Stimulating   Balancing   Relaxing

BODY SYSTEMS

PROPERTIES > USES

NERVOUS SYSTEM
■ ■ ■ □ ■ ■ ■

antispasmodic, tonic > neuralgia, stress

ENDOCRINE SYSTEM
■ ■ ■ ■ ■

causes sweating, hormone like, temperature reducing, stimulates secretions > bile, good woman's oil

CIRCULATION AND IMMUNE SYSTEM
■ ■ ■ ■ □ ■ ■ ■

acts on the bone marrow stimulates blood renewal, astringent, lowers blood pressure, decongestant > varicose veins

SKIN, MUSCLES and BODY TISSUES
■ ■ ■ ■ □ ■ ■ ■

antiinflammatory, antiseptic, cell generator > baldness, back ache, ulcers, wounds

RESPIRATORY SYSTEM
■ ■ □ ■ ■ ■

antiseptic > catarrh

DIGESTIVE SYSTEM
■ ■ ■ □ ■ ■ ■

stimulant > diarrhoea

URINARY SYSTEM
■ ■ ■ ■ □ ■ ■ ■

balances urine flow and urine retention, diuretic > bed wetting, cystitis , kidney scars

REPRODUCTIVE SYSTEM
■ ■ ■ ■ ■ ■

abortive, emmenagogue > fibroids, ovaries, period problems, prolapse

CAUTIONS

Avoid in pregnancy and with young children powerful oil.

BOTANICAL FAMILY

Compositae : this family is generally soothing especially for the skin and digestion.

Plant: distilled flowering heads : sweet spicy camphorous aroma : middle note.
Used in Scotland to ward off evil spirits. Considered an 'all healing' plant.

Chemical constituents may include:

■ bornyl acetate

■ isoartemisia, camphor, thujone

■ chamazulene, caryophyllene, germacrene, dihydroazulene

■ achilline

□ 1.8-cineole, caryophyllene oxide

■ limonene, α-pinene,β-pinene, sabinene, camphene, myrcene

■ borneol, terpinen-4-ol, cadinol

■ eugenol

YLANG YLANG
Cananga odorata

■ esters		15.0%
■ aliphatic aldehydes		0.1%
□ ketones		0.1%
■ sesquiterpenes		40.0%
□ remainder		14.4%
□ acids		yes
■ monoterpenes		0.4%
■ alcohols		20.0%
■ phenols,phe. ethers		10.0%

Stimulating   Balancing   Relaxing

BODY SYSTEMS	PROPERTIES > USES
NERVOUS SYSTEM ■■■■■■■	aphrodisiac, antispasmodic, balancing, calming, sedative, tonic > anxiety, depression, fear, panic, shock
ENDOCRINE SYSTEM □□■■	regulates adrenaline flow >
CIRCULATION AND IMMUNE SYSTEM ■■■□■■	lowers blood pressure, balances sebum production > slows heart beat
SKIN, MUSCLES AND BODY TISSUES ■■■□■■	antiseptic > possible skin irritation, stimulates hair growth
RESPIRATORY SYSTEM ■■□■	calming > slows breathing pace
DIGESTIVE SYSTEM □■■□■■	stimulates secretions > diabetes, gastric, intestinal infections
URINARY SYSTEM	
REPRODUCTIVE SYSTEM ■■■■■■■	stimulates ovaries and testicles > frigidity, impotence
CAUTIONS	Use with care can cause headaches and nausea.
BOTANICAL FAMILY	Annonaceae.

Small tree: distilled flowers : sweet heavy exotic aroma : base note.
In Indonesia wedding beds are strewn with the flower petals. Used extensively in perfumes.
Chemical constituents may include:

■ methyl benzoate, <u>benzyl acetate,</u> benzyl benzoate, <u>geranyl acetate</u>

■ farnesol, geraniol, <u>linalool</u>, benzyl alcohol

■ β-caryophyllene, cadinene, farnesene, <u>germacrene</u>, humulene

■ methyl eugenol, eugenol, safrole, p-cresyl methyl ether

□ pinenes

3 | Indices and References

Therapeutic Properties Index for the Oils

A

abortive *10, 14, 26, 65, 74, 84, 89*
air antiseptic *21, 35, 66, 77, 79*
anaesthetic *52, 53, 54*
analgesic *8, 9, 16, 21, 22, 28, 29, 30, 31,*
32, 33, 34, 38, 39, 41, 42, 49, 53, 56,
59, 62, 67, 68, 69, 72, 73, 74, 83
antiaging *11, 43, 58, 59*
anticoagulant *22, 24, 26, 33, 46, 58*
antidepressant *41*
antifungal *4, 5, 7, 10, 14, 15, 19, 20, 24,*
27, 33, 40, 41, 42, 43, 44, 45, 49, 53,
55, 58, 59, 60, 61, 62, 63, 64, 69, 70,
72, 73, 74, 77, 78, 79, 81, 83, 86
antiinflammatory *1, 3, 9, 12, 16, 18, 20,*
27, 29, 30, 32, 33, 36, 39, 40, 42, 44,
45, 46, 50, 53, 54, 55, 58, 61, 64, 66,
69, 71, 72, 75, 76, 79, 81, 82, 83, 86,
87, 89
antimicrobic *52, 63*
antioxidant *6, 19, 21, 32, 33, 34, 49, 60,*
85, 86
antiseptic *1, 2, 3, 4, 6, 7, 8, 9, 10, 11, 12,*
13, 14, 15, 17, 19, 21, 22, 23, 24, 25,
26, 27, 28, 29, 30, 31, 33, 34, 36, 37,
38, 40, 41, 42, 43, 44, 45, 46, 47, 48,
49, 51, 52, 53, 54, 55, 56, 57, 58, 60,
61, 62, 63, 64, 65, 66, 67, 68, 69, 70,
71, 72, 73, 74, 75, 76, 78, 80, 81, 82,
83, 85, 86, 87, 88, 89, 90
antispasmodic *1, 3, 4, 7, 8, 10, 12, 13, 14,*
16, 18, 19, 20, 21, 22, 23, 24, 27, 30,
32, 33, 34, 36, 37, 38, 39, 40, 42, 43,
46, 47, 49, 50, 51, 52, 53, 57, 59, 60,
62, 65, 67, 71, 72, 74, 75, 79, 81, 82,
85, 86, 89, 90
antiviral *1, 2, 3, 4, 5, 7, 8, 12, 19, 21, 22,*
25, 27, 28, 35, 41, 42, 43, 46, 47, 49,
53, 55, 56, 62, 63, 64, 66, 70, 72, 73,
74, 77, 78, 82, 83, 86
aphrodisiac *4, 8, 15, 17, 19, 34, 37, 38, 49,*
59, 64, 69, 71, 73, 76, 77, 88, 90
astringent *6, 13, 14, 19, 23, 32, 36, 54, 55,*
58, 64, 72, 75, 76, 77, 84, 89

B

bactericidal *1, 2, 3, 4, 5, 7, 8, 10, 11, 13,*
15, 16, 17, 18, 19, 20, 21, 22, 23, 24,
27, 30, 31, 32, 33, 36, 40, 41, 42, 43,
44, 45, 46, 48, 49, 51, 52, 53, 55, 56,
57, 58, 59, 60, 61, 62, 63, 64, 66, 67,
68, 69, 70, 71, 72, 73, 74, 76, 77, 78,
79, 80, 81, 82, 83, 85, 87
balances menstrual cycle *82*
balancing *14, 15, 16, 23, 33, 34, 42, 49,*
51, 53, 59, 64, 71, 82, 89, 90
balm *14*
bleeding stems *80*
blood pressure lowers *1, 4, 11, 20, 27, 36,*
40, 42, 43, 46, 49, 50, 59, 61, 72, 75,
81, 89, 90
blood pressure raises *21, 36, 53, 65, 69, 72,*
74, 78, 85
bone marrow acts on *89*
breast decongestant *30*

C

calming *1, 2, 6, 7, 9, 11, 12, 16, 18, 20, 26,*
27, 28, 29, 32, 33, 35, 37, 40, 41, 42,
43, 45, 47, 48, 49, 50, 54, 55, 58, 59,
60, 63, 64, 66, 71, 76, 80, 88, 90
carminative *61, 62, 64, 65*
cell regenerator *11, 32, 33, 42, 47, 58, 59,*
63, 64, 81, 89
cheering *6, 34, 42, 58, 60, 63, 66, 71*
clarifying *43*
cortisone like *69, 79*

D

decongestant *1, 2, 3, 6, 8, 11, 13, 14, 15,*
16, 17, 20, 23, 25, 26, 28, 29, 30, 31,
33, 36, 39, 40, 41, 42, 43, 46, 48, 54,
56, 61, 64, 66, 68, 69, 71, 72, 74, 75,
76, 81, 82, 83, 89
deodorant *6, 20, 60, 73*
diuretic *6, 8, 11, 13, 14, 15, 23, 26, 30, 33,*
35, 36, 38, 39, 43, 44, 45, 49, 54, 55,
62, 64, 66, 67, 69, 71, 72, 74, 76, 78,
80, 82, 84, 85, 89

E

emmenagogue *4, 17, 18, 19, 36, 42, 49,*
55, 57, 62, 65, 71, 72, 74, 75, 81, 82,
88, 89
euphoric *22*

Therapeutic Uses Index for the Oils

A

abscesses *78*

aches and pains *8, 31, 41, 56, 67, 69, 70, 80, 88*

acne *4, 13, 14, 16, 21, 41, 44, 45, 56, 60, 63, 64, 75, 79, 85, 86, 87, 88*

addiction *49*

adrenal cortex *4,33,75*

adrenal glands *69*

aerophagy *62*

afterbirth *4, 42, 85*

aging skin *32, 43, 76*

agitation *7, 52*

allergies *4, 16, 27, 40, 50, 69, 82*

amenorrhoea *16, 17, 18, 20, 30, 38, 55, 72, 75, 82, 88*

anaemia *8, 11, 18, 50, 85*

anger *10*

angina *8, 30, 34, 50*

anorexia *11, 19, 22, 30, 63, 82*

antibodies *56*

anxiety *3, 4, 9, 11, 32, 33, 40, 42, 46, 47, 58, 80, 85, 90*

appetite depressant *64*

appetite stimulant *18, 38, 46*

arteries *15, 17, 24, 31, 44, 45, 49, 66*

arteriosclerosis *39, 72*

arthritis *2, 6, 12, 13, 14, 15, 25, 26, 27, 31, 34, 42, 43, 49, 67, 68, 69, 75, 82, 85, 87, 88*

asthma *18, 20, 25, 26, 27, 28, 30, 32, 36, 53, 56, 68, 69, 71, 75, 80, 83, 85*

athlete's foot *25, 33, 41, 44, 45, 55, 64, 81, 83*

B

back pain *18, 29, 34, 89*

bad breath *22*

balances blood sugar *6*

baldness *14, 20, 89*

bedsores *55*

bedwetting *72, 89*

bee stings *50*

bereavement *76*

bile *7, 10, 16, 17, 24, 42, 47, 50, 52, 54, 61, 71, 72, 74, 77, 82, 86, 89*

birth delivery *37*

bites *29, 83*

bleeding *19, 33, 43, 46, 67, 71, 88*

blood sugar *25*

blood vessels *11, 23, 33*

boils *7, 16, 30, 36, 43, 56, 67, 72, 83, 85*

break down fats *47*

breast congestion *33*

breast inflammation *32*

breathing *19, 30, 32, 37, 49, 50, 90*

broken veins *71*

bronchial dilator *81*

bronchial secretions *85*

bronchial spasms *37, 86*

bronchitis *1, 2, 3, 5, 8, 10, 11, 13, 14, 15, 21, 23, 24, 26, 28, 30, 31, 32, 34, 36, 39, 41, 42, 43, 49, 53, 54, 55, 56, 59, 60, 61, 62, 63, 65, 66, 67, 68, 69, 70, 71, 74, 78, 79, 80, 83, 86*

bronchopneumonia *73*

brown patches *43*

bruises *8, 36, 41, 49*

bunions *81*

burns *16, 33, 42, 56, 83*

C

calluses *81*

calms digestion *16, 46*

calms excitement *2*

calms yet alerts *41*

cancer *10, 32*

candida *25, 27, 33, 42, 72, 73, 74, 78,79, 83, 86*

capillaries *23, 53, 71*

carbuncles *32, 85*

cardiac *6, 8, 30, 36, 41, 63, 77*

catarrh *4, 6, 8, 10, 13, 14, 24, 25, 26, 28, 31, 32, 34, 36, 39, 41, 43, 46, 49, 56, 65, 67, 68, 72, 74, 75, 76, 83, 89*

cellulite *15, 23, 30, 38, 43, 44, 45, 74*

cervix *63*

chest infections *36, 55*

chicken pox *7, 25, 27, 70*

chilblains *8, 11*

childbirth *19, 20, 21, 24, 30, 34, 37, 38, 42, 53, 57, 63, 85, 86*

chills *61*

chlorosis *21*

cholesterol *20, 34*

chronic conditions *14, 73, 82, 87*

circulation *6, 44, 45, 49, 57, 58, 66, 68, 72, 74, 75, 78, 85*

gastritis *3, 4*
genital herpes *56, 74*
genital infections *32*
gingivitis *71, 75*
gives strength *30, 37*
glands tonic *19, 22*
glandular fever *55, 70*
gnats *25, 53*
gonorrhoea *25, 76*
gout *4, 11, 18, 39, 43*
greasy hair *13, 20, 39*
grief *36, 50*

H

haemorrhage *25*
haemorrhoids *1, 13, 14, 20, 23, 33, 55, 57, 59, 64, 76, 83*
hair growth *57, 90*
hair loss *15, 75, 85*
hangover *34*
hayfever *36*
headaches *17, 24, 26, 28, 35, 42, 43, 49, 50, 54, 75*
hearing *34*
heart regulation *4, 49, 50, 51, 76, 90*
heart stimulant *52, 53, 57, 65, 72, 86*
hepatitis *4, 11, 53, 55, 69, 72*
herpes *7, 12, 21, 25, 27, 42, 50, 53, 55, 70*
hiccoughs *4, 82*
HIV *56*
Hodgkin's Disease *21*
hot flushes *74*
hysteria *50, 83*

I

immune system *1, 5, 10, 11, 32, 55, 60, 62*
impetigo *33, 78*
impotence *21, 51, 53, 57, 69, 71, 76, 90*
indigestion *7, 8, 10, 22, 24, 30, 34, 36, 50, 52, 61, 69*
indigestion nervous *58, 60*
infected pus *17*
infections *1, 2, 12, 30, 35, 55, 71, 77, 78, 81, 90*
infertility *11*
insects *16, 19, 27, 64, 65, 84*
insomnia *16, 17, 18, 38, 40, 42, 43, 47, 50, 70*
intestines *82, 90*
irritability *17, 18, 23*
irritable bowel syndrome *12*

irritations *18, 46, 52, 62, 90*
itching *6, 76, 83*

J

jaundice *11, 18, 33, 53, 71, 75*
jealousy *71*
joints painful *28, 38, 63*

K

kidney stones *11, 30, 33, 36, 38, 39, 43*
kidneys *4, 11, 14, 21, 26, 52, 76, 82, 89*

L

lactic acid *44, 45*
laryngitis *25, 27, 52, 53*
laxative *49, 82*
leucocytes *16, 62*
leucorrhoea *6, 7, 13, 14, 15, 19, 25, 26, 32, 36, 42, 55, 56, 65, 67, 74, 85*
liver *2, 3, 4, 8, 11, 17, 18, 21, 23, 26, 33, 35, 38, 43, 44, 45, 47, 50, 51, 52, 53, 54, 58, 59, 65, 70, 71, 74, 75, 77, 86, 87, 88*
liver stimulant *58*
loneliness *6*
loose skin *64*
lower back spasms *34*
lumbago *68, 76*
lungs *22, 23*
lymph circulation *15, 69, 80*

M

maggots *81*
malaria *4, 25, 78*
malignancies *74*
mature skin *20*
measles *25*
memory loss *21*
meningitis *74*
menopause *17, 18, 20, 23, 59*
menstrual *11, 16, 17, 18, 19, 22, 23, 30, 36, 38, 42, 50, 53, 82, 89*
mental fatigue *22, 39, 53*
metabolic rate *47*
midges *41*
migraine *4, 16, 18, 25, 35, 42, 52, 53, 54, 72*
milk decrease *53*
milk increase *4, 10, 24, 30, 37, 44, 45*
mosquitoes *21, 25, 81*
moths *21*
motor nerves *52, 57*
mouth infections *83*

mouth ulcers *61, 83*
mucous decongestant *38*
mucous irritant *77*
mucous membranes *11, 62*
mucous stimulant *19, 48*
multiple sclerosis *36, 69*
muscle aches *28, 31, 41, 49, 67, 69, 70*
muscle cramps *1, 29*
muscle relaxes *37, 40*
muscle toner *21*

N

nausea *19, 34, 50*
neckache *29*
nephritis *25, 32, 52, 53*
nervous exhaustion *26, 33, 51, 54, 60, 63, 75, 78*
nervous tension *13, 14, 61, 81*
nervous trembling *53*
nervous system *3, 53, 72*
neuralgia *8, 15, 18, 19, 21, 26, 33, 34, 57, 62, 75, 76, 82, 89*
neuritis *18, 41, 74*
nightmares *43*

O

obesity *38, 43, 61*
obsessional *32, 49*
oedema *30, 38, 74*
oily skin *14*
osteoarthritis *22*
otitis *49, 53, 72*
ovarian function *23*
ovaries *51, 53, 69, 79, 83, 89*

P

palpitations *30, 50*
palsy *74*
pancreas *2, 3, 6, 8, 23, 25, 33, 38, 51, 59, 74, 88*
panic *20, 90*
paralysis *8, 30*
parasites *2, 7, 17, 30, 36, 51, 56*
para-sympathetic nerves *44, 45, 49*
peace inducing *59*
periods heavy *89*
periods irregular *22, 23, 89*
periods none *16, 17, 18, 20, 75, 82, 88, 89*
periods painful *16, 17, 18, 33, 49, 75, 82, 89*
periods scanty *20, 57, 72, 88, 89*

pests *44, 45*
phlebitis *13, 14, 20, 40, 42, 59, 64*
plaques *3*
pleurisy *23, 66*
pmt *23, 33, 59, 71, 82*
pneumonia *2, 3, 5, 25, 56*
poison *84*
polio *3, 21*
postnatal depression *20, 32*
prolapse *89*
prostate *2, 3, 17, 23, 38, 39, 53, 56, 78*
protective shield *88*
pruritus *7, 15*
psoriasis *6, 7, 11, 13, 16, 18, 38, 42, 69, 74, 86*
psychoses *49*
puffy skin *20*
pulmonary artery *3, 55*
purification *10, 19, 22, 75, 82*
pyorrhoea *23*

R

radiography burns *42, 56, 59, 83*
rashes *1, 16, 29, 53*
Raynaud's Disease *8, 21, 30, 33, 42, 57, 71, 72*
respiratory system *81*
renal TB *78*
revitalising *59, 79*
rheumatism *2, 6, 8, 12, 13, 14, 15, 16, 22, 23, 26, 27, 31, 33, 34, 36, 39, 41, 43, 46, 49, 56, 57, 59, 60, 62, 61, 68, 72, 75, 79, 80, 82, 84, 85, 86, 88*
rheumatoid arthritis *3, 8, 21, 74, 78*
rhinitis *39, 41, 49, 52, 53, 63, 75*
rhinopharyngitis *36*
ringworm *41, 53, 55, 67, 83*

S

sadness *6, 22*
saliva *19, 21*
scabies *67*
scabs *27*
scalp problems *10*
scarlet fever *25*
sciatica *26, 38, 52, 53, 67, 76, 82*
scurvy *46*
seasickness *34*
sebum *14, 15*
senses *81*
sensitivity *88*

sexual obsession *49*
sexual stimulus *55*
shingles *7*
shocks *18, 24, 83, 90*
sight *34*
sinusitis *4, 13, 21, 26, 29, 36, 40, 42, 46,*
    49, 52, 53, 54, 56, 63, 66, 68, 69, 70,
    75, 86
skin care *11, 37, 73*
smell sense restorer *4*
solar plexus *29*
soothing *51*
sore throat *27, 29, 56, 86*
sores *26, 27, 29*
spasms bowel *1, 4, 21, 82*
spasms gastric *1, 10, 29, 82*
spasms intestinal *1, 10, 78, 82*
sperm count *37*
sperm production *69*
spleen *17, 65, 71*
spots *9, 42, 56, 83*
sprains *57*
stiffness *38, 63*
stings *29*
strangury *38, 39*
strength and courage *30*
stress *13, 16, 35, 46, 54, 80, 85, 88, 89*
stretch marks *37, 47*
surgical scars *18*
sweaty feet *23, 83*
swellings dissolve *30, 36, 72*

T

TB *15, 21, 23, 42, 59, 66, 71, 78, 83, 86,*
    87
tears stimulant *19*
tension *81, 88*
threadworms *4*
thrush *7, 43, 55, 74, 83*
thymus *79*
thyroid *11, 21, 49, 55, 79*
tired legs *44, 45*
tissue regenerator *10*
tonsillitis *7, 25, 33, 86, 87*
toothache *8, 10, 16, 19, 21, 34, 49, 52, 57,*
    74
travel sickness *4, 53*
trembling *52, 53, 74*
tropical infections *3*
typhoid *25*

U

ulcers *6, 11, 14, 16, 21, 26, 32, 55, 56, 74,*
    89
ulcers gastric *4, 11, 16, 43, 49, 52, 53, 56*
urethritis *67, 86*
uric acid *4, 38, 82*
uterine haemorrhage *33*
uterine muscles *37*
uterus *4, 63, 69*

V

vagina *63*
vaginal infections *37*
vaginal secretions *22, 27*
vaginitis *86*
varicose veins *1, 13, 20, 33, 34, 42, 59, 64,*
    76, 83, 89
vasodilatory *44, 45, 49*
veins *3, 88*
vertigo *4, 10, 49, 50, 58*
verrucas *43, 86*
vomiting *52, 53, 54*

W

warming *22,62,66*
warts *19, 43, 84*
wasp stings *4, 50*
weakness *55, 80*
white corpuscles *55, 85*
whooping cough *4, 23, 30, 67, 70, 72, 83*
woman's oil *89*
worms *4, 9, 52, 53, 62, 82, 85*
wounds *6, 11, 15, 16, 21, 24, 27, 29, 32,*
    40, 42, 54, 67, 71, 74, 75, 82, 83, 85,
    89
wrinkles *30, 32*

Y

yellow fever *3, 53*

Chemical Constituents Index for the Oils grouped in Chemical Families

■ Esters

angelates *18*
benzyl acetate *17, 19, 37, 90*
benzyl benzoate *19, 37, 90*
bornyl acetate *17, 31, 36, 38, 40, 66, 67, 69, 72, 74, 75, 79, 80, 84, 87, 89*
bornyl butyrate *17*
bornyl caproate *66*
bornyl propionate *66*
butyrates *18*
cis- carvyl acetate *54*
trans- carvyl acetate *54*
cinnamyl acetate *19*
citronellyl acetate *27, 50, 58, 71*
citronellyl butyrate *27*
citronellyl citronellate *27*
citronellyl formate *33*
coniferyl benzoate *6*
coniferyl cinnamate *6*
dihydrocarvyl acetate *54*
fenchyl acetate *3, 4, 72*
geranyl acetate *11, 20, 22, 29, 35, 42, 43, 46, 49, 50, 51, 58, 59, 60, 63, 71, 78, 86, 90*
geranyl formate *33, 63*
geranyl hexanoate *63*
geranyl isobutyrate *63*
lavandulyl acetate *42*
linalyl acetate *3, 4, 7, 20, 22, 37, 40, 41, 42, 48, 49, 51, 58, 59, 60, 62, 74, 75, 78, 85, 86, 87*
menthyl acetate *29, 52, 53*
methyl anthranilate *37, 46, 47, 59*
methyl benzoate *90*
methyl cinnamate *4*
methyl jasmonate *37*
methyl myrtenate *36*
myrrholic ester *55*
neoisomenthyl acetate *65*
neryl acetate *20, 43, 50, 59, 60, 71*
neryl formate *63*
octyl acetate *32*
trans- pinocarvyl acetate *48*
propionates *18*
sabinyl acetate *75*
terpinen-4-yl acetate *23*
terpinyl acetate *38, 43, 48, 49, 56, 69, 70, 75, 78, 85*

α- terpinyl acetate *23, 25*
terpinyl butyrate *56*
terpinyl valerate *56*
tiglates *18*
vetiverol acetate *88*

■ Aliphatic Aldehydes

2- butanal *55*
caproaldehyde *66*
caryophyllenal *20*
citral *7, 33, 35, 42, 43, 44, 45, 46, 47, 49, 50, 58, 60, 63, 69, 81*
citronellal *27, 34, 35, 43, 47, 50, 61, 63, 69, 73*
decanal *43, 47, 61*
decylaldehyde *22, 31*
geranial *12, 29, 34*
hexanal *74*
isovaleraldehyde *28, 56*
lauraldehyde *31*
neral *12, 29, 71*
nonanal *43*
octanal *43, 61*
sinensal *35, 47*
undecanal *58*

■ Ketones

α- atlantone *15*
γ- atlantone *15*
camphor *3, 17, 20, 22, 36, 40, 41, 42, 48, 72, 74, 75, 77, 78, 79, 84, 85, 87, 89*
carvone *9, 10, 22, 24, 54, 61, 72, 81*
cryptone *66, 69*
curzerenone *55*
dihydrocarvone *8, 10, 24, 54, 87*
fenchone *30, 68, 74, 84*
gingerone *34*
α- ionone *61*
isoartemisia *89*
isomenthone *52, 53*
isopatchoulenone *64*
isopinocamphone *36*
trans- isopulegone *65*
isothujone *84*
jasmone *59*

Sesquiterpenes

Lactones and Coumarins and Furan Derivatives

Others

eugenol methyl ether *5*
isoeugenol *21*
methyl chavicol (estragole) *2, 3, 4, 30,*
    36, 67, 68, 74, 82, 87
methyl eugenol *3, 4, 71, 90*
methyl hexyl ether *20*
myristicin *8, 57*
safrole *8, 19, 57, 90*
thymol *5, 47, 48, 60, 62, 74, 77, 78, 85,*
    87
thymol methyl ether *5*

NOTE:

caproaldehyde	=	*hexanol*
decylaldehyde	=	*decanal*
eugenol methyl ether	=	*methyl eugenol*
methyl chavicol	=	*estragole*

References

1   *Musajo, L., Rodighiero, G., Caporale, G.* (1954). The photodynamic activity of the natural coumarins. Bull. Soc. Chim. Biol. 36, 1213-1224 XXX

2   *Zheng, G.Q., Kenney, P.M., Lam, K.K.T.* (1992). Anethofuran, Carvone and Limonene: Potential Cancer.

3   *Achterrath-Tuckerman, U. et al.* (1980). Pharmacological investigations with compounds of chamomile. V. Investigations on the spasmolytic effect of compounds of chamomile. Planta Medica 39, 38-50.

4   *Salamon., I.* (1992). Chamomile production in Czecho-Slovakia. Focus on Herbs 10, 1-8.

5   *Szelenyi, I. et al.* (1979). Pharmacological investigations with compounds of chamomile. III. Experimental studies of the ulcerprotective effect of chamomile. Planta Medica 35, 218-227.

6   *Melegari, M. et al.* (1988). Fitoterapia V.LIX. n.6.

7   *Low, D. et al.* (1974). Planta Medica V.26, 184-189.

8   *Albert-Puleo, M.* (1980). 1. Ethnopharmacol. 2, 337-344.

9   *Davis, P.* Aromatherapy, An A-Z, 135.

10 *Deans, S. et al.* (1987). Intl. J. of Food Microbiol. 5. 165-180.

11 *Martindale.* (1972). The Extra Pharmacopeia. The Pharmaceutical Press. 26th Edition.

12 *Knobloch, K. et al.* (1989). J. Es. Oil, Research 1, 119-128.

13 *Lis-Balchin, M., Deans, S. and Hart, S.* (1994). Paper: 25th International Symposium on Essential Oils, Grasse, France.

14 *Maruzella, J.C.* (1960). Soap Parfum Cosmet. 33, 835-7.

15 *Yousef, R.T. and Tawil, G.G.* (1980). Pharmazie 35, 698-701.

16 *Asre, S.* (1994). Chemical Composition and Anti-microbial Activity of some Essential Oils, M.Sc. Thesis, Macquarie University, Sydney, Australia.

17 *Torii, S., Fakuda, H., Kanemoto, H., Miyanchi, R., Hamanzu, Y., and Kavaski.* (1988). In Perfumery 107-20.

18 *Mabey, R.(Ed.)* (1988). The Complete New Herbal. Elm Tree Books, London.

19 *Dew, M.J.* (1984). Br. J. Clin. Pract., 38, 394-8.

20 *British Herbal Pharmacopoeia.* (1983). 148.

21 *Shafran, I., Mauer, W., and Thomas, F.B.* (1977). New England. J. Med. 296, 694.

22 *Maruzella, J.C. and Liguori, L.* (1958). J. Am. Pharm. Ass. 47, 250.

23 *Maruzella, J.C.* (1960). Soap Parfum Cosmet., 33, 835-7.

24 *Tisserand, R.,* The Essential Oils Safety Data Manual, 89.

25 *Ohloff, G.* (1994). Scent and Fragrances, Springer Verlag.

26 *Betts, T.* (1994). Aromatherapy Quarterly, 19-22.

27 *Taddei, I., et al.* (1988). Fitoterapia V. LIX, n. 6.

28 *Tisserand, R.,* The Essential Oils Safety Data Manual, 96.

Bibliography

Beckett, S., Herbs to Soothe Your Nerves, Thorsons, 1977.

British Herbal Pharmacopoeia, British Herbal Medicine Association, 1983.

Culpeper, N., Culpeper's Complete Herbal, W. Foulsham and Co. Ltd, 1952.

Davis, P., Aromatherapy An A-Z, C.W.Daniel, 1988.

Duke, J.A., Handbook of Medicinal Herbs, CRC Press, Boca Raton, 1985.

Franchomme, P., Livre Quatrième, Eléments de Matière Médicale Aromatique Fondamentale.

Franchomme, P., Phytoguide I, International Phytomedical Foundation, La Courtête, France, 1985.

Franchomme, P. and Pénoël, D., L'Aromathérapie Exactement, 1990.

Grieve, M., A Modern Herbal, Penguin, 1982.

Grosjean, N., Aromatherapy from Provence, C.W.Daniel, 1993.

Guenther, E., The Essential Oils, Vol. 1-6., Van Nostrand, New York, 1948.

Jackson, J., Aromatherapy, Dorling Kindersley, 1987.

Lis-Balchin, M., The Chemistry and Bioactivity of Essential Oils, Amberwood, 1995.

Lautie, R. and Passebecq, A., Aromatherapy: The Use of Plant Essences for Healing, Thorsons, 1982.

Lawless, J., The Encyclopaedia of Essential Oils, Element Books, 1992.

Lawless, J., Aromatherapy and the Mind, Thorsons,1994.

Lawrence, B.M. Essential Oils, Allured Publishing Co., Wheaton, USA, 1978.

Kroch, A.&C.A., Guide to the Medicinal Plants of the United States, Quadrangle, The New York Times Book Co., 1973.

Mabey, R.(Ed.), The Complete New Herbal, Elm Tree Books, London, 1988.

Maury, M., Marguerite Maury's Guide to Aromatherapy, C.W. Daniel, 1989.

Mills, S.Y., The Essential Book Of Herbal Medicine, Penguin Arkana, Harmonsworth.

Metcalfe, J., Herbs and Aromatherapy, Webb and Bower, 1989.

Phillips, R., Wild Flowers of Britain, Pan, 1977.

Ody. P., The Herb Society's Complete Medicinal Herbal, 1992.

Percival, A., Aromatherapy - A Nurses Guide, Amberwood, 1995.

Price, S., Aromatherapy for Common Ailments, Gaia Books, 1991.

Price, S., Aromatherapy Workbook, Thorsons, 1992.

Price, S. and Price, L., Aromatherapy for Health Professionals, Churchill Livingstone, 1995.

Ranson, F., British Herbs, Penguin, 1949.

Rich, P., Practical Aromatherapy, Parragon Book Services, 1994.

Ryman, D., The Aromatherapy Handbook, Century, 1984.

Secondi, O., Handbook of Perfumes and Flavors, Chemical Publishing Co., New York, 1990.

Sellar, W., The Directory of Essential Oils, C.W.Daniel, 1992.

Stead, C., The Power of Holistic Aromatherapy, Javelin Books, 1986.

Le Strange, R., A History of Herbal Plants, Angus and Robertson, 1977.

Tisserand, M., Aromatherapy for Women, Thorsons, 1990.

Tisserand, M., Stress: The Aromatic Solution, Hodder and Stoughton, 1996.

Tisserand, R. and Balacs, T., Essential Oil Safety, A Guide for Health Care Professionals, Churchill Livingstone, 1995.

Valnet, J., The Practice of Aromatherapy, C.W. Daniel (English Version), 1982.

Westwood, C., Aromatherapy - A Guide for Home Use, Amberwood, 1991.

Westwood, C., Aromatherapy - For Stress Management, Amberwood, 1993.

Wildwood, C., Aromatherapy, Element Books, 1991.

Worwood, V.A., The Fragrant Pharmacy, Macmillan, 1990.

Worwood, V.A., The Fragrant Mind, Doubleday, 1990.

Wren, R.C., Potter's New Cyclopedia of Botanical Drugs and Preparations, C.W.Daniel, 1988.

Glossary

Abortive: capable of inducing abortion.

Adrenaline: secretion from adrenal glands that speeds up heart, constricts small blood vessels and increases metabolic rate.

Adrenal cortex: three zoned centre of adrenal glands situated just above each kidney.

Aerophagy: swallowing of air.

Amenorrhoea: absence of menstruation.

Anaesthetic: causes loss of feeling.

Analgesic: deadens pain.

Anaphrodisiac: reduces sexual desire.

Anorexia: loss of appetite, eating disorder.

Anticoagulant: counteracts coagulation.

Antidepressant: helps alleviate depression.

Antifungal: combats fungal infections.

Antiinflammatory: calms inflammation.

Antioxidant: delays oxidation

Antiparasitic: destroys parasites.

Antimicrobial: destroys pathogenic micro-organisms.

Antispasmodic: eases spasms and convulsions.

Antiseptic: destroys and prevents the development of microbes.

Antiviral: inhibits growth of viruses.

Aphrodisiac: increases sexual desire.

Arteriosclerosis: thickening of arteries.

Arthritis: inflammation of joints.

Astringent: causes constriction of tissues.

Bactericidal: destroys bacteria.

Balm: soothing medicine or application.

Cardiac: pertaining to the heart.

Carminative: relieves flatulence.

Catarrh: inflammation of mucous membranes causing increase of secretion.

Cellulite: accumulation of toxins in body tissue in the form of fat.

Chemotype: the same botanical species occurring in other forms due to different conditions of growth such as climate, soil, altitude and so on.

Chlorosis: a rare form of anaemia.

Cholesterol: a common animal sterol, precursor of many hormones, excess in the body can lead to the formation of gall stones and to impaired arteries.

Coagulation: transformation of liquid to soft semisolid state.

Cortisone: a corticosteroid used to treat various conditions in particular arthritis, certain allergies and diseases of connective tissues.

Cystitis: bladder inflammation.

Decongestant: reduces congestion.

Deodorant: agent that counteracts body odour.

Dermatitis: inflammation of the skin; many causes.

Diarrhoea: frequent passing of loose stools.

Diuretic: aids production of urine, increases flow.

Dopamine: dopamine is a chemical produced by the brain – lack of dopamine causes Parkinsonism.

Dysmenorrhoea: painful menstruation.

Emmenagogue: induces or assists menstruation.

Euphoric: exaggerates sense of well being.

Expectorant: helps to clear mucous from the respiratory system.

Febrifuge: combats fever.

Galactagogue: increases milk production.

Genito-urinary: referring to both the genital and reproductive systems.

Gingivitis: inflammation of the gums, swelling and bleeding.

Gout: a condition of excess uric acid in the blood.

Glossary

Hallucinogenic: causes visions or delusions.

Haemorrhoids: piles, dilated rectal veins.

Haemostatic: arrests bleeding.

Heartwood: centre of tree trunk.

Hepatic: relating to the liver.

Herpes: virus infection causing blisters and clusters of deep seated vesicles.

Hormone: a product of living cells which controls body functions.

Hypertension: high blood pressure.

Hypertensive: raises blood pressure.

Hypnotic: causing sleep.

Hypotension: low blood pressure.

Hypotensive: lowers blood pressure.

Insecticide: repels insects.

Insomnia: inability to sleep.

Leucocyte: white blood cells that fight infection.

Leucorrhoea: white discharge from the vagina.

Lipolytic: breaks down fatty tissues.

Lumbago: painful rheumatic affliction of the muscles and fibrous tissues in the back.

Menopause: the normal cessation of menstruation, a life change for women.

Menorrhagia: excessive menstruation.

Metrorrhagia: uterine bleeding outside of normal cycle.

Mucolytic: breaks down mucous.

Narcotic: induces sleep, intoxicating can be poisonous in large doses.

Nervine: strengthens nervous system.

Nephritis: inflammation of the kidneys.

Neuralgia: stabbing pain along a nerve path.

Neurotonic: tonic to the nervous system.

Neurotoxic: poisonous to the nervous system.

Oedema: painful swelling caused by fluid retention under the surface of the skin.

Oestrogen: a hormone triggered from the pituitary gland that controls female reproductive processes.

Olfaction: sense of smell.

Otitis: inflammation of the ear.

Palpitation: uneven or rapid heart beats.

Parasiticide: prevents and destroys parasites such as fleas, lice and so on.

Phototoxic: causes skin to become sensitive to sunlight.

Pituitary gland: gland attached to base of brain that controls production of body hormones.

Prostatitis: inflammation of the prostate.

Pruritus: itching.

Psoriasis: a skin disease exhibiting red patches and silver scaling.

Regulator: helps balance and regulate the body functions.

Relaxant: relieves tension and stress.

Renal: pertaining to the kidney.

Rhinitis: inflammation of nasal mucous membranes.

Rhizome: an underground stem lasting more than one season.

Sedative: reduces functional activity, calming agent.

Strangury: painful and slow urination due to spasms of the urethra and bladder.

Thrush: fungal infection (candida)

Tonic: strengthens body functions.

Vasoconstrictor: narrows blood vessels.

Vasodilator: dilates blood vessels.

Vermifuge: expels intestinal worms.

Vesicle: small sac or blister containing fluid.

Vulnerary: helps wounds heal.

Amberwood

OTHER BOOKS AVAILABLE FROM AMBERWOOD PUBLISHING ARE:

AROMATHERAPY - *A guide for home use by Christine Westwood*. All you need to know about essential oils and using them.
£1.99   ISBN 0 9517723 0 9.

AROMATHERAPY - STRESS MANAGEMENT - *A guide for home use by Christine Westwood*. Covering the use of essential oils for everyday stress-related problems.
£3.50   ISBN 0 9517723 6 8.

AROMATHERAPY - FOR HEALTHY LEGS & FEET - *A guide for home use by Christine Westwood*. A guide to the home use of essential oils for the treatment of legs and feet.
£2.99   ISBN 1 899308 04 0.

AROMATHERAPY - A NURSES GUIDE *by Ann Percival* SRN. The ultimate safe lay guide to the natural benefits of Aromatherapy. Including recipes and massage techniques for many medical conditions and a quick reference chart.
£3.50   ISBN 1 899308 04 0.

AROMATHERAPY - A NURSES GUIDE FOR WOMEN *by Ann Percival* SRN. Concentrates on women's health for all ages. Including sections on PMT, menopause, infertility and cellulite.
£2.99   ISBN 1 899308 12 1.

AROMATHERAPY - THE ESSENTIAL BLENDING GUIDE *by Rosemary Caddy* Bsc Hons, ARCS MISPA. An exciting way to use essential oils in the home. The book gives well tried recipes for effective blends of essential oils for 50 common ailments.
£9.99   ISBN 1 899308 24 5.

AROMATHERAPY LEXICON - *The Essential Reference by Geoff Lyth and Sue Charles*. This informative Lexicon is remarkable for its simplicity and makes understanding Aromatherapy easy. This form of reference will give endless pleasure to beginners as well as practised Aromatherapists.
£4.99   ISBN 1 899308 15 6.

AROMATHERAPY - SIMPLY FOR YOU *by Marion Del Gaudio Mak*. A new updated edition of the simple and thorough guide to Aromatherapy that has been so successful. Easy reference chapters explain everything from purchasing and storage of essential oils to the beneficial effects to be had from their use.
£2.99   ISBN 1 899308 10 5.

AROMATHERAPY - THE CHEMISTRY & BIOACTIVITY OF ESSENTIAL OILS *by Dr Maria Lis-Balchin*. With a comprehensive list of the Oils and scientific analyses. Includes a section on the sense of smell and the history of Aromatherapy.
£5.99   ISBN 1 899308 21 0.

ALL YOU EVER WANTED TO KNOW ABOUT VITAMINS *by Dr. Leonard Mervyn*. Dr Mervyn explains why we need extra vitamins, and what can happen to our long term health if we don't get them in adaquate quantities, and who is most at risk from deficiency.
£6.99   ISBN 1 899308 22 9.

INDIAN MEDICINE - FOR THE IMMUNE SYSTEM - *Echinacea by Dr Desmond Corrigan* BSc(Pharms), MA, Phd, FLS, FPSI. An intriguing account of the history of the plant called Echinacea and its power to influence the immune system.
£2.99   ISBN 0 9517723 7 6.

HERBAL MEDICINE FOR SLEEP AND RELAXATION *by Dr Desmond Corrigan* BSc(Pharms), MA, Phd, FLS, FPSI. A guide to the natural sedatives as an alternitive to orthodox drug therapies, drawing on the latest medical research, presented in an easy reference format.
£2.99   ISBN 1 899308 07 5.

GINKGO BILOBA - ANCIENT MEDICINE *by Dr Desmond Corrigan* BSc(Pharms), MA, Phd, FLS, FPSI. (New Edition) Improved memory, circulation and concentration are associated with Ginko Biloba and explained in this book.
£2.99   ISBN 1 899308 04 0.

NATURAL TASTE - HERBAL TEAS - *A guide for home use by Andrew Chevallier* BA, MNIMH. Contains an impressive compendium of Herbal Teas gives information on how to make it, its benefits, history and folklore.
£3.50   ISBN 0 9517723 8 4.

NATURAL MEDICINE - HERBAL FIRST AID - *A guide for home use by Andrew Chevallier* BA, MNIMH. A beautifully clear reference book of natural remedies and general first aid in the home.
£3.50   ISBN 0 9517723 5 X.

PLANT MEDICINE - *A guide for home use by Charlotte Mitchell* MNIMH (New Edition).This book provides the perfect guide, explaining both the properties of plant medicines and how to use them. As more and more people seek alternatives to modern drugs, interest in natural plant remedies grows.
£3.50   ISBN 1 899308 13 X.

HOW GARLIC PROTECTS YOUR HEART *by Professor Edzard Ernst* MD PhD. Used as a medicine for over 4500 years, this book examines the latest scientific evidence supporting Garlic's effect in reducing cardiovascular disease, the Western World's number one killer.
£3.99   ISBN 1 899308 08 3.

WOMEN MEDICINE - VITEX AGNUS-CASTUS *by Simon Mills* MA, FNIMH. The story of the herb that has been used for centuries in the treatment of women's problems. The author examines the medical properties on symptoms relating to menstruation and the menopause.
£2.99   ISBN 0 9517723 3 3.

FENG SHUI - *A guide for home use by Karen Ward*. Simple tips on 'Power of Place' and effects of environment on health.
£2.99   ISBN 1 8993082 3 7.

Amberwood

INSOMNIA - DOCTOR I CAN'T SLEEP *by Dr Andrian Williams* FRCS. Written by one of the worlds sleep experts, Dr Williams explains the phenomenon of sleep and sleeping disorders and gives advice on treatment. With 25% of the adult population reporting difficulties sleeping - this book is essential reading for many.
£2.99   ISBN 1 899308 09 1.

ARTHRITIS & RHEUMATISM - *The Sufferers Guide by Dr John Cosh* FRCP MD. It is a complete guide to understanding the painful and sometimes progressive disease, whilst offering many useful tips to alleviate the symptoms.
£4.95   ISBN 1 899308 17 2.

CANCER-HERBS IN HOLISTIC HEALTH CARE *by Dr J Walker.* Cancer in its various forms can give rise to a wide range of unpleasant symptoms, either due to the disease itself, or its treatment, or the fear associated with it. In this book we read of the drugs commonly used in the conventional treatment of cancer and their many possible side effects..
£15.99   ISBN 1 899308 28 8.

HERBAL MEDICINE FOR CHILDREN *by Frances Hambly.* A simple easy to understand guide for parents who want to know about herbal medicine and appropriate natural treatment for children.
£6.99   ISBN 1 899308 30 X.

HERBAL MEDICINE FOR DOGS *by Mary Boughton.* So many dog owners would love to know how to use herbs to help their pets stay healthy. The author, Mary Boughton, is a manufacturer of vetinary herbal medicine and has been involved with herbs and dogs all of her life..
£5.99   ISBN 1 899308 25 3.

HERBS FROM THE BIBLE *by Patricia Armstrong.* The author delves into the biblical text to find out what people thousands of years ago used as medicines, as flavourings for food, as dyes for there clothes and perfume. Her knowledge of the Bible combined with her understanding of medicinal plants make fascinating reading.
£9.99   ISBN 1 899308 29 6.

AROMATHERAPY - THE BABY BOOK *by Marion Del Gaudio Mak.* An easy to follow guide to massage for the infant or child.
£3.99   ISBN 1 899308 18 0.

AROMATHERAPY THE PREGNANCY BOOK *by Jennie Supper* RM RN MGCP. Midwife Jennie Supper has many years experience of bringing new people into the world. Her book deals with making the birthing process pleasurable by using beautiful aromas for calming tension and natural pain relief.
£5.99   ISBN 1 899308 20 2.

PHYTOTHERAPY 50 VITAL HERBS *by Andrew Chevallier.* The most popular medicinal herbs with uses and advice written by an expert.
£6.99   ISBN 1 899308 19 9.

CADDY BLENDING CALCULATOR

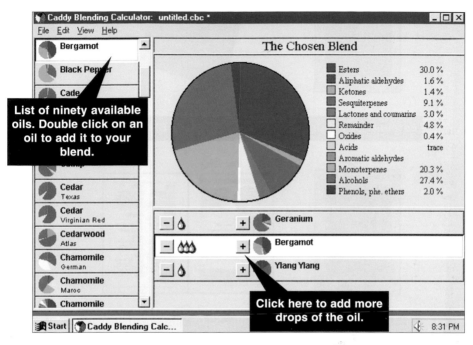

| Caddy Blending Calculator: untitled.cbc * | _ □ × |

File   Edit   View   Help

The Chosen Blend

■ Esters	30.0 %
■ Aliphatic aldehydes	1.6 %
□ Ketones	1.4 %
■ Sesquiterpenes	9.1 %
■ Lactones and coumarins	3.0 %
□ Remainder	4.8 %
□ Oxides	0.4 %
□ Acids	trace
■ Aromatic aldehydes	
■ Monoterpenes	20.3 %
■ Alcohols	27.4 %
■ Phenols, phe. ethers	2.0 %

Bergamot
Black Pepper
Cade

List of ninety available oils. Double click on an oil to add it to your blend.

Cedar — Texas
Cedar — Virginian Red
Cedarwood — Atlas
Chamomile — German
Chamomile — Maroc
Chamomile

Geranium
Bergamot
Ylang Ylang

Click here to add more drops of the oil.

Start — Caddy Blending Calc...   8:31 PM

- •*Enables Creative Blending*
- •*90 Essential Oils to Blend*
- •*Step by Step Instructions*
- •*Blends in Living Colour*
- •*Make-up of Blend at a Glance*
- •*Print on Client's Record Sheet*

An excellent companion to 'Essential Oils in Colour' the Caddy Blending Calculator opens up a new world of exploration. It uses the 90 Oils in the book and at a glance you can see the chemical make-up of any blend.

You can explore your trusted blends and see their chemical make-up. You can adjust your blends to suit individual needs. Print your blend for your records.

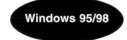 **Windows 95/98**

 October Pen SOFTWARE

CD-ROM

For further information:
Tel: +44 (0)1803 835290
E-mail: mail@ccprofiles.co.uk   Website: www.ccprofiles.co.uk

Teaching Materials

Guildford College
Learning Resource Centre

Please return on or before the last date shown.
No further issues or renewals if any items are overdue.
"7 Day" loans are **NOT** renewable.

1 0 NOV 2005

Class: 615.321 CAD

Title: Essential oils in colour

Author: Caddy, Rosemary.

For further information:

Tel: +44 (0)1803 835290

E-mail: mail@ccprofiles.co.uk   Website: www.ccprofiles.co.uk

145380